I Am Joe's Heart (Attack)

TYLER + VIRNA
HAVE A GOOD
READ.
YOU CAN READ IT
BUT YOU CAN'T
UN READ IT

Joe Mauro

JOE MAURO

PAGE PUBLISHING, INC.
New York, NY

First originally published by Page Publishing, Inc. 2017

ISBN 978-1-68409-989-4 (Paperback)
ISBN 978-1-68409-990-0 (Digital)

Printed in the United States of America

My Simple Story of a Profound Adventure

I would like to thank my immediate family, especially my father; for without his help, I never would have had this heart attack. He did put me in his gene pool. I would like to thank my wife for proof-reading, and my brothers and sister, for their editing and advice on this book. My mother, for feeding me all the sausage and great cold cuts I have eaten all my life, and especially for the crispy potatoes she would cook with pork fat, or whatever other fat was available. I would like to give special thanks to my brother Jaime, who predicted that a family disaster such as this would occur with one of the siblings. The only problem is that the patient didn't die... yet. Also my deceased brother Johnny should be mentioned, since he gave me and my whole family its first experience in dealing with disaster, sickness, and death. Johnny died in 1970 at the age of sixteen. He is greatly missed by all of us and taught us a lot about living, by dying. I would like to thank my extended family. Without whose help, I wouldn't have had all that great greasy food we always consumed at our family reunions. I would like to thank my employer, the weather company I worked for, as well as all their clients; for without them, there would not have been enough anxiety and stress in my life to bring me to the point of a myocardial infarction—which I shall from now on refer to as simply a heart attack, because it is much too long a word to write and much too complicated to spell. Seriously, I would like to thank Chris and Tracey, my kids (whom, from now on, will be called the little stress makers), for not panicking when I had my heart attack. Lastly, I would like to thank the medical community, without whose help and constant flip-flopping their thoughts on healthy foods as often as I change my underwear, I—and probably ten million other people—might not have had heart attacks. Think of the billions of dollars that have been made on these so-called extra heart attacks, more on this later.

Joe

Prologue

How do I start this discussion, a book on *I Am Joe's Heart "Attack"*?

I guess that, as we go through this thing called life, we have to answer some pretty deep and complex questions, such as, Why are we even here? Is there a god, or isn't there a god? Is there life on other planets? Does the light in the refrigerator go out when the door is closed? When all is said and done, there are questions we will never have an answer for. I guess my question for now is, Why did I have a heart attack? Not that I am even worried about it; I am more pissed off about it. I did everything the doctor's suggested, even when they changed their minds I tried to accommodate them. Butter bad, I quit butter and went to margarine. Uh-oh, margarine is worse, so I went back to butter. I was right on track. Incidentally, my brother Jason, who is still in perfect health, once ate an entire stick of butter when he was in grammar school. It didn't kill him; he had the trots for a couple of days, but no heart problems.

I am a corporate meteorologist, a weatherman. I tell people what the weather will be. I, along with all my peers, am wrong from time to time. Hey, show me a human being that has never been wrong. Our problem is that our forecasts (same as a prognoses) go public every day. Therefore, we take a lot of abuse for erroneous forecasts. I say that doctors are often wrong when it comes to their prognoses (same as forecasts), but they don't get the abuse that weathermen do because they don't go public.

I have experienced some war stories dealing with the medical community. Some doctors are as incorrect as stock analysts and worse than weather forecasters when diagnosing problems. Just a word about the importance of my forecasts as a meteorologist—unlike the television weatherman saying, "partly sunny and warm," airline meteorologists have to be extremely accurate because like diagnoses in the medical community, lives are at stake. We had to deal with corporate aviation. We had the responsibility of getting aircraft from place to place in the safest possible way. We had a myriad of weather calculations to consider—such as, ground conditions, where and when thunderstorms could affect a flight, we also had to account for upper level winds and turbulence, as well as legal alternates the planes can divert to in the event of bad weather—at all times in communication with the pilots, assuring they had enough fuel onboard for all the possible changes if our calculations were in error. Even with small planes, many could die in weather related accidents.

All health care is unbelievably expensive, even when erroneous diagnoses are made. I was in one hospital for three days; the bill was around $35,000. I wish as a meteorologist I could make that kind of money even when I am wrong. Unlike meteorologists, whose forecasts are public, health-care workers' forecasts are private mostly for fear of frivolous lawsuits.

I wish there was a study performed as to how many times the medical community has contradicted itself with advice that you should follow in order to be healthy. I can't keep up with it. It starts with diets, don't eat fat, then it's okay to eat fat. Then you can eat certain types of fat. We had the butter fiasco in the prologue. They say drinking will kill you, but now it is okay to have moderate drinks of wine. One day vitamin C is great for you; the next day it will make your platelets too sticky. It's known that vitamin C cures colds, but wait a minute, there is no proof it cures colds. Eat carbohydrates, but Dr. Atkins says eat all the meat and fat you want. Then Dr. Atkins dies a fat person because the diet only works over a short period of time. Try the sugar-buster diet; don't eat any carbs. We have to exercise for an hour three times a week, but no twenty-minute sessions equal an hour when we exercise. There are many differences of opinion concerning artificial sweeteners. I personally can't keep up with all the different advice I hear about getting and staying healthy. There are also many obviously stupid contraptions on the market. My physical education degree tells me that much more checking should be done before this junk is offered for sale. Shopping channels should have more pride in themselves and a moral obligation to their customers to sell a good, effective product. I am glad I made it through my first heart attack, and in no way am I pissed off at my local doctors and nurses. They did a great professional job, and they saved my life. But as a whole, the medical community should get their act together because people often listen to their conflicting advice, on what is healthy and what is not. If they are not sure of something don't say or do anything at all.

Sometimes it seems that money has become more important to the medical community than good service. I hate to bring this up, but I think someone has to say it: we have become too acceptable of the medical community for their costly wages and many times poor results. I don't refer to local doctors who earn an honest living helping patients as best they can. Doctors worry about frivolous lawsuits all day long in their private practices. Hypothesize for a while. This is just my opinion, and it may or may not be true. Let's call it food for thought. Suppose a cure for cancer was found tomorrow. In fact, in my hypothesis, this might already have happened. What if someone designed a car that got five hundred miles per gallon of gas. Surely, some big oil company would buy this idea and bury it because they would care less about the common good, and more about their financial situation. I feel the same thing could happen if a cure for cancer was found. First of all, we would not need all these cancer researchers anymore; they would have to be directed to other pursuits. Many practitioners are getting rich on cancer research with very little in the way of results. We have spent trillions on cancer research both from charity and government, yet the bottom line is that with cancer, if you can't excise it, we will die eventually from it. Having spent trillions on research, the long and short of it is, if you get liver or pancreatic cancer, there is little hope. We haven't mentioned how the government would be affected by a cancer cure. What would happen to Medicare, Medicaid, and Social Security if as a result, people started living much longer lives? Should we trust the government or the medical community with this question? There is a lot of greed out there. I think I will burn in hell and die of a strange disease very quickly if this book gets published. Again, just food for thought.

Contents

CHAPTER 1

The Early Years

To begin with, my name really is Joe, and this is a true story of what happened to me. While all the facts are true, anything that has to do with opinions are mine and mine alone. The medical community, the government, or anybody else should not hold my friends and family accountable for my views, and I think many of you will agree and see my side of things.

I should briefly elaborate on my childhood and tell you that I was one of five siblings—who, early in life, lived on Staten Island, New York. At one time, my father had five children, a wife who had no gainful employment, other than being a good mother, and only made $80 a week. But I will save all this superfluous information for my autobiography (or biography), whichever comes first, if this book is successful. I will, from time to time, go my own way and interrupt the story occasionally to tell of some family and friends, but that's all for now. All you need to know at this point is that since November 1, 1956, I was already predestined by my genes (please refer to the introduction). I was destined to have a heart attack. I guess the only question was when.

Let's talk about the contributing factors. Since I was young, I didn't know I was going to have a heart attack. As a matter of fact, I knew I wouldn't. I did have my fair share of fun and games as a child.

I remember taking part in bicycle races and winning them as early as 1964. I once won a race, turned back to laugh at the kid I just beat, and promptly ignored his yelling and finger-pointing (he tried to save my life). I crashed into a parked car, chipping my front tooth (which remains chipped even today), and cutting my ear. I really was not a fantastic athlete, but I did participate in little league. I went to summer school at PS 41 a school in Staten Island NY and did nothing but play all kinds of games—such as, softball, war, dodge ball, buck buck—and never once had any chest pains.

We moved to Connecticut before I could even pronounce it in 1968. I was in sixth grade at the time (after being left back, which is another story I will save for my possible later book). I joined the middle school soccer team, and though my memories from that are hazy, I recall playing in many soccer games. I was always active, never a skinny child. I was not morbidly obese either, everybody said I was "husky."

When I was in seventh and eighth grade, my gym teacher started a walkers club. This was a club where we would all walk around a circular parking lot that measured one-tenth of a mile around. Our gym teacher, our resident Neanderthal man—and by the way, he really looked like one—ran the program. We would use our "study hall" time to walk, and since I was never one who enjoyed studying too much, I would walk. He had a ten-mile club, a fifty-mile club; of course, I would always get into the one hundred–mile club. Still, though, no sign of heart problems, but the genes were getting ready for a surprise.

It was in these years when I first had a stressful and anxious period. It occurred in the late summer and early fall period of 1970 when my oldest brother Johnny began coughing a lot. It seemed like, for weeks, he just had this nasty hacking cough. I must emphasize that I am telling this story from my perspective, a thirteen- to fourteen-year-old kid who didn't know at the time what was going on.

Ever since, I never had the courage to ask what actually happened; there was nothing anyone could do about it now, anyway. After a while, a week or two, my mother took Johnny to the doctor and evidently had many tests performed. Around October or so, we were told that he had pneumonia, which I thought was serious but not too bad a thing. That same night was my first clue that something was seriously wrong.

My dad came home from work, and my mother said out loud to my dad, "Do you know what John has?

My dad guessed, "Pneumonia?"

My mother thought for a minute, hesitated, and said yes.

At this point, I think she knew it was leukemia. Just the way she acted suggested something was wrong. They went into their bedroom and had a short talk right after dinner. From this point, unusual things were beginning to happen. For example, about a week after this, we saw Johnny going out with his friends walking down the street on a cold morning, with no hat on. My mother had always been a stickler about wearing hats in cold weather. Here, my brother with pneumonia didn't have to? Something wasn't right. There were frequent trips to the hospital where my brother would remain for anywhere from one day to a week or so. But through October and November, whenever we saw him, he would always be coughing. From mid-October on, he always had tissues with him because he would be coughing then spitting up blood.

One Saturday morning (perhaps mid or late November), I was working on my paper route. This is where I would bike to deliver my papers to homes in a very affluent town, Madison. Some of the people were millionaires, and I am sure I delivered to a few of them, but they were so generous that when the papers were ninety-five cents a week, some would give me a dollar but do you think they were so generous they would give me a tip? No, they would say, "Take the nickel off of next week's bill." I was about two miles away from home, and I had a flat tire. My father was coming home from a business trip (he traveled a lot), and he saw me. Dad stopped the car—boy, was I glad to see him—and asked how everything was. I said that Mom took Johnny to the hospital last night. He had trouble breathing, a problem he had several times. Doctors would drain fluid from around his lungs, and he would be okay. At that point it was, "Bye-bye, Dad." He left me to walk my broken bike home. I never blamed him for this and suspected, with more confidence that something was seriously wrong.

Johnny was in the hospital through early December. Mom and Dad said the pneumonia was serious, but still I never thought that death was in the equation. Johnny had a few bad days in early December, but from my last talk with Mom around December 7 or so, I got the impression that he was doing a little better for the last day or two. I remember this day as though it were yesterday. All our relatives came to our house on Wednesday, December 9. Being from New York City, these relatives never came up on weekdays, and this was a Wednesday. But I remember Aunt Marie, Uncle Frank, and Grandpa most specifically. They said Johnny looked real sick. I thought that he had a few bad days three or four days ago, and that may have made him look bad; but again, I thought he was doing better. So I wasn't too worried at this time. We ate dinner without Mom and Dad as they frequently would be at the hospital. After dinner, I caught my Aunt Marie crying as she was washing the dishes. Now I was getting worried.

The final blow occurred about 10:00 p.m. at night. My brothers and sister were in bed. The phone rang, and I heard my Aunt Marie say, "Is it over yet?" Yikes… this is serious… But it was not over at this point. I couldn't sleep, knowing what was about to occur. At about 1:00 or 2:00 a.m., Mom and Dad came home and basically said it's all over. Dad took me aside and told me that my brother had leukemia and died. They told us it was not pneumonia but cancer of the blood.

Johnny did not want us to know. I don't know how many relatives did know. I was too shocked to be upset. I really pitied my siblings Jaime, Jason, and Jill for the ordeal that was to come to them in six or seven hours. I was lucky. I got hints throughout the day before, and they hadn't. This was a family disaster that would take years to get over. I don't think we are totally over it yet, and it happened over thirty years ago. I really feel bad for Mom and Dad... losing a son is hard enough but some maintain that Mom and Dad handled the situation poorly by keeping us in the dark. I maintain and always will that there was no right or wrong way to handle this. Johnny wanted to keep it a secret; anything handled improperly was unavoidable. My parents were forty years old, and their son died. Everyone was devastated by this event. There are more details I could get into, but my big brother dying is as sad as it gets. Let's just leave it at that.

After Johnny's death, all the teachers in the school were very nice and understanding. One teacher actually asked me during a test if I was doing okay, which I thought was very nice of her, and I assured her I was fine. My friends didn't say a lot, I think no one knew what to say, except for one classmate. He was a nice person but a greaser-type a guy in my class.

I remember seeing him in the hall, and he asked, "How are you doing?"

I tried to tough it out by saying something like, "Okay he was only my brother."

He looked me in the eyes and said, "I know you truly miss him," as if it was all right.

Then he walked away—a truly insightful thing to say considering how young he was. I liked him, and though we were never best friends, we knew each other throughout high school. A sad thing about him was that he was killed in a traffic accident about ten years after this. Let's move on to a lighter subject and go on to high school. Not too many middle school kids get heart attacks, and I was no exception.

CHAPTER 2

High School

Finally, in high school, I was a guy—a real man, a mature adult. My time had finally come. Back in my day, when I attended high school (in the early 1970s), there were two types of people: the greasers and the jocks. Actually, in high school, I couldn't decide what I was. I guess I was some sort of hybrid. Through high school, I was on the football team for two years, wrestling team for four years, and the track team for four years. But I always seemed to hang around with the greasers. This must have driven my coaches crazy because greasers and jocks mixed about as well as oil and vinegar.

When I was a freshman, the freshman football coach recruited me to play for the freshman football team. I never had a lot of interest in football up to this point, but I thought it looked like fun. Being about 190 lbs., I was easily the biggest freshman; and if it wasn't for a big black guy who was part of the Madison, CT ABC program, I would have been the biggest man on the varsity team. The head coach of the varsity team did not really want a big football team, but he did want a fast, tough, well-disciplined team. While playing football, I realized rather suddenly that my name changed from Joe to Mauro. I couldn't have been more wrong about how much fun I thought football would be.

"Mauro, do this…" "Mauro, do that…" "Mauro, you are dogging it…" "Mauro, hit harder…" "Mauro, my grandmother could run faster…"

I wanted to tell him that his grandmother would be a great asset to the team because it seemed she could jump higher, run faster, and hit harder than anyone on the team. I really didn't say this. He would have killed me before I had a chance to get a heart attack.

Football by itself was hard enough. But as I said before, I was the biggest guy on the team, so you can guess where the coach wanted me to play: on the line, in the trenches, worse than that, it was on the offensive line. You couldn't even use your hands, you just blocked people and watched them beat the shit out of you. Yeah, real fun! The coaches warn you that on the line there is no glory; you will never get much ink in the newspapers. As a lineman, you were the one responsible for winning and losing games. In the long run, it became obvious to me that we were only responsible for losing games not winning them. The running backs were responsible for winning games. Another great duty we had as freshman football players is that if we were good enough, we would play on the scrimmage team against the junior varsity team. This basically meant that the older kids (sophomores and juniors) could legally beat the crap out of you to make you tougher and more experienced to play with the older kids. I was not great for the first few weeks of football, but after a while, I caught on and started to get better. You will find out in this book that I was never and will never be a natural at anything physical. I just simply did not have it in my genes—as we know, I had better plans with my genes, why waste them on sports. I did, however, persevere and worked hard and succeeded to some degree.

Another advantage of playing football is the weather. I don't care how cool the summers were in those days, we had this thing that football players do called double sessions. This is what always turned out to become the hottest week of summer (the week before school starts), when you would much rather be at the beach we had to "play" football. In Madison, Connecticut, we lived in a town right on the waters of Long Island Sound and had a private beach. I could have been at the beach or playing with my friends (even greaser friends). As a matter of fact, I would rather have had hot needles in my eyes or bamboo shoots stuck under my fingernails or even got water boarded than go through double sessions in football. The coach would pick this "best week of summer" to spoil it for everyone on the team. This is where you would get to enjoy practice two times a day. We would practice once from 9:00 a.m. till noon, the other from 3:00 p.m. to 6:00 p.m., or something like that—just enough to screw up your entire day. These torture segments went from Monday to Saturday. Sunday, you couldn't enjoy because most of us were too busy licking our wounds from the previous six days. Just in case you did have some free time to kill during this period, you could always memorize your fifty-page playbook. This would actually be a good thing because you couldn't move. These long practices didn't save you from doing extra laps or wind sprints. By the way, I would love to wring the neck of the guy who invented wind sprints. As I started out saying at the beginning of this paragraph before I got sidetracked, no matter how cool the summers were up to double session's week, you could bank on the fact that the hottest week of summer was always the double session's week. So we did all the crap above when the temps were in the midnineties' and humidity was through the roof. I am sure that if you look at the national weather service records for the last week of August in the early 'seventies when I was playing football, you can see a spike in the temperature graph.

To digress for a moment, I'll get back to football, I think. Things like the above are things that just affect me. I pity those closest to me (friends, neighbors, relatives, etc.) because they are stuck in my sphere of influence, something on the order of being near a black hole and can do nothing about it. I don't just drag me down; I drag everyone down, call it my bad karma. I'm sure you've heard the expression, "If it wasn't for bad luck, I'd have no luck at all."

An example of this is that real estate has gone through the roof, constantly increasing in value since the beginning of time. All economic forecasters, real estate experts, and the like, predicted this trend would continue forever, and it did, until Joe bought a house. The real estate market still hasn't recovered. When I go shopping and I am waiting in the checkout line, I apologize to people in back of me because my line will always be the slowest, not because of me, but because I am in the line. For some reason I always happen to pick the slowest people in front of me. This has happened many different times to me, but the only common thread I can find is that I am in the line.

Getting back to football for a moment, I mentioned the oppressive heat that we always had to deal with. Usually, the oppressive heat would last until a certain date. Let's call this date for the sake of argument, October 15. On that date and from that date on, there would be nothing else but frigid cold. Again, check the weather records. I don't think I ever played or practiced football when the temperature was between forty and eighty; it was always above or below these numbers. My mother used to do the laundry for me when I was in high school. We have to understand that she had four kids and a husband (a very demanding one), so she couldn't focus all her laundry attention on me. She had three other kids and a husband to shop for, to cook for, to drive around town, to entertain, to take to doctor and dentist appointments, music lessons, friends' houses, and birthday parties, etc., etc., etc. I think you get the picture. She had a lot to do. You can again check the weather records if you want to, but I bet that it rained every Monday in the early 'seventies after October 15. Why? I'll tell you: it would not dare rain before October 15 because it would make it too cool and comfortable for our football practices. (The coach would not like that too much.) But after it got cold, the weather gods—or football gods, or whoever—knew that my mom would wash our football stuff on weekends. Of course, the temperature would be in the midthirties and raining every Monday, so my football uniform would be muddy, sandy, and very cold during practice. What was worse was that for the next four days, it would take me at least ten minutes just to get used to the uniform before I could put it on. It was grimy, gritty, and cold, and you did not feel like moving in this thing until about the time practice was over. That sucked. But as we know, what does not kill us makes us stronger—or at least, I thought it did. But still no heart pains yet; the only pain in my life now was football.

As a freshman, I got to eventually start at offensive right tackle. Then I got better and better and played junior varsity football by midseason. By late season, I was dressing up for varsity games and even played in a couple of blowout games.

As a sophomore, I was a starter on the junior varsity and varsity teams. Again, at 190 lbs., I was, of course, the largest person on the team. The ABC kid finally graduated, and again I had every bit as much "fun" as I had as a freshman. In the fifth game of the season, I had a little problem, however. The other team we were playing had these two 300 lb. bookends playing on their team. They were on the defensive line, and one of these 300 lb. gorillas was always right across from me. Guess who had the "privilege" of blocking them—me, of course. The day after this game, I started getting a rather strong pain in my lower left abdomen. This was not the heart attack yet; that pain had to be in the chest. It turned out that I had a hernia—or, in other words, a great excuse to sit out the rest of the football season. Boy, did I miss playing football (right). After that, I finally got the courage to tell the coach that my football career was over—a decision, I must say, I have never regretted.

After my freshman season, this coach did manage to talk me into joining the wrestling team. This was a brand-new sport not only for me but for our whole high school. Being new to the sport, I had no clue what it was about. I would like to say I wrestled my first year, but I think the reality of the situation was that I was simply a tool, much like a mop, used to clean the mats between the 167 lbs. weight class and the heavyweights. The whole team, again because they were new to the sport, kind of sucked, but we did have one or two standouts. To say one was a muscle-bound middle linebacker from the football team is an understatement. He was big and strong, mean, tough, and probably lost 30 lbs. to get to the 158 lbs. class. He was an animal. I don't know what his record was, but I recall a time when he was losing a match and decided he had no other option than to bite a huge boil on the back of one of his opponents. I was not so gifted. I don't know what my record was as a freshman, but I know that when your coach says the famous line, "Just don't get pinned," he really didn't expect much from me. I think the word *fish* would have described my wrestling very well during my freshman year.

After winning one of our matches as a freshman—not me, but the team, because I am pretty sure I mopped the mat that night—our coach felt it was the right time to tell a wrestling story. It goes like this.

One night in the state championship finals in the heavyweight class, there were two wrestlers. One was a senior and had won the heavyweight crown the past three years. The other was a junior, who had never won the heavyweight crown but had won at the 185 lbs. class the year before. They were both very talented, well-decorated veterans of the sport. The underdog, the junior, had a conversation with his coach before the match. The coach reminded him that "we were in our gym"; the championships happened to be in his own high school with all his hometown fans. He added that he was faster, stronger, and (he felt) smarter than the senior. Out of a total of over one hundred bouts, the senior won about 99 percent of them by using his special maneuver called the pretzel hold. The coach said in the four years he had known this senior, no one has ever escaped from this and always had gotten pinned from it.

He said to his junior, "You could beat this senior, but don't get caught in this pretzel hold."

During the first two rounds of this match, the kids both fought well, and the score was 3 to 2 in favor of the senior. As the third round started, his kid (the junior) got caught in this pretzel hold. The coach ran to the locker room, cursing and knocking down everything in sight. Garbage cans, lockers, towels, equipment were flying across the locker room. Then the coach just sat there. After a few seconds, he heard the crowd roaring and clapping. Remember, this was a hometown crowd; something good must have happened to his kid. As the coach left the locker room, he saw the referee raising the hand of his kid. He had won the state title. When the hoopla was all over, the coach took the kid to his office and asked him how he beat the pretzel hold. The young man said that when he got in this hold, he thought it was over; he was literally tied up like a pretzel. He went on and said that he eventually saw these two things dangling in front of him.

Then he said to his coach, "It is amazing how fast you can move when you bite yourself in the balls."

I wrestled in the 185 lbs. weight class, which meant that when the season started in December, the weight limit was 185 lbs. but by the time the season ended with the sectionals and states, the weight class would be 189 lbs. to allow for the kids to grow somewhat. I feel that I did myself a big favor wrestling in the 185 lbs. class—the reason being that if you were in good shape and were even a hint athletic, you would lose some weight to wrestle in a lower-weight class. If you were strong and lost weight, you would have a better chance winning against a lighter person. Most high school kids who weighed 180 lbs. were just fat. So if you had your wits about you, lose weight and wrestle lighter kids. Only if you were lazy would you stay at the 185 lbs. weight class. I was real good at being lazy. Also, the majority of kids from fourteen to eighteen years old really were averaging from 120 to 160 lbs. This made just by sheer numbers the middle weight classes very competitive. You also had your morbidly obese people that the coach would recruit to be the heavyweight, not to wrestle so much but just to sit on people. God knows that a 250 lb. high school kid could not be athletic at all; that is how they got so fat in the first place. This breed was too fat and lazy to lose any weight at all. And tucked in there between the average kids with some athletic ability (160 lbs. or less) and the fat ones (200 lbs. or more) were the one or two people just right for the 185 lbs. class. Trust me, I was not a great athlete, but I worked hard. I got my ass kicked the first couple of years, but if you want to succeed in wrestling, go to the 185 lbs. class, where most of the kids were losers—at least in those days. Generally, the kids were too fat to wrestle at a lower weight and too skinny to compete with the very fat heavyweights.

I mopped the mats the first couple of years, but by virtue of my weight (185 to 189 lbs.), I ended up doing very well by my senior year. By then, even though I was outweighed by about 15 lbs., I was quick, smart, and strong and could go on forever because I was in very good shape. I even looked up some moves in the library (such as home run takedowns) that actually pinned some opponents in a stunning manner. This even shocked my coaches because they were wondering where I learned these moves. They know it didn't come from them. My senior year, I had done better than anyone else in my high school ever did before me. I was the third best wrestler in the state in the 189 lbs. class (even though I weighed about 170 lbs.). The funny thing is that I, in the previous week, pinned the guy who eventually got second place in the state.

I could expound on the fact that in high school, I was on the track team for four years and actually was one of the co-captains my senior year, but in reality, I never ran an event in high school. I threw the shot put and discus, which I don't think is really "cardiovascular" enough to prevent heart attacks. I did have a coach in track with a great sense of humor. When I was a freshman or sophomore, the coach almost gave the captain of the track team a heart attack.

It was April Fools' Day, I think, the coach came out of his office acting all kinds of pissed off. When he saw the captain walking toward him, he took out his starter's gun (which is nothing more than a blank gun with a plugged barrel) and shot the captain, who crumpled almost to his knees and held his stomach, thinking the coach really flipped out and shot him. Both people were laughing when it was all over. The coach would always do things like this to keep the team loose. The real story here is that both people had fun with it; no one sued anyone, and for that reason alone, I feel the world has lost something it once had. People are so suit conscious and politically correct that many practical jokes and good experiences are missed because people fear the courts. If this happened today, a great guy like the coach would probably be in jail, or at least banned from coaching, for an otherwise harmless event that both people had fun with.

My only real regret in high school was not joining the golf team, not that it would have done a lot for my heart, but it is a good activity in which you can participate until you are well into your seventies. Try playing football or wrestling that long. I don't think we see a whole lot of people throwing shot puts and discuses at that age either. I didn't go out for the golf team because many thought you were a sissy if you did. I guess it seems like an easy sport, until you really try it. This was in the days when I actually cared what everyone thought.

I did spend a lot of time during my summers and vacations and weekends running on the streets, keeping in shape for whatever sport I was participating in. So all in all, through high school, I had no health problems. But I will say again: the storm was brewing. This is because I feel genes and heredity override most of the good stuff you can do physically.

CHAPTER 3

The College Years Round 1

On to college, or should I say, college the first time around. Learning is so much fun that I had to go twice. Or was I so stupid that I had to go twice? I'll explain now why I went to college two times. When I got out of high school, I thought I wanted to be a physical education teacher. I went to Southern Connecticut State College, which was a fairly well known teachers' college, especially physical education teachers' college. Also, rumor had it that there was a 7–1 ratio of girls to guys, another thing that made this college hard to overlook (I'm not bragging, but I got my share). I have to admit I had a real good time at Southern, and the years I had there I wouldn't trade for anything. Getting a PE degree at SCSC was fairly easy as well. They had special classes for PE majors that were very, very easy. One example was chemistry. There was a course just for physical education majors, which was well known as kiddy chem. I did have a small problem during my first class at this school. I had an Oriental teacher in my first class, which just happened to be a US history class. Imagine this, a new student in strange new surroundings (like me), not really knowing the ropes, or anyone else at this school, and the teacher starts taking attendance…

"Mr. Krouse…" "Here…" "Mr. Larkins…" "Here…" "Mr. Larson…" "Here…" "Mr. Marlo…" "Here…" (I said, "Here." I was

Mauro, but with an Oriental teacher, Marlo was close enough for me.) Then the teacher said "Mr. Mauro…" Oh, boy, what do I do now. I remember being real apologetic and such, but I blacked the rest of it out of my mind. I wish Mr. Marlo would have not skipped class that day.

After about three years at SCSC, I decided that I really did not want to teach. But at this point, I really had no choice but to stick it out and finish my four years and get my bachelor of science degree in physical education. I was very fortunate, though, in that my father was a very strong believer in education. Sure, I was going to be ticked off at him because in several years, he was going to have a heart attack and put it in my family history, but I didn't know this yet. My mom and dad knew I have always had an interest in weather and in fact told me if I had a deep interest in weather, I should pursue it and get a degree in meteorology. He insisted that there was no time like the present to do this. So I tried to find a good meteorology school. This is no simple task, as there are not too many strong undergraduate schools in this program. I finally applied and got accepted at the University of Oklahoma (I only heard of this school because of its football team, but what the heck). I didn't like playing football, but I sure loved watching it.

My mother is the main reason I became interested in weather. When I was a child, I loved snow more than anything. I also was evidently an unruly young child. In church, I would yell at the top of my lungs, "Ding a ling a ling, I'm the priest"—which, I am sure, embarrassed my mother. She knew how to push my buttons, though, when she had to. She would tell me that she was going to call the weatherman and tell him to not let it snow tomorrow. Since I am talking about my childhood, one of my other stories will follow.

When I was young, my mother would take me and my three brothers shopping. Can you imagine a lady with four kids shopping in the first place? Anyway, she told me to pull up my zipper, to which

I replied, "Okay, Mommy." It was hot in that store, so I would pull it down the first chance I got.

Later, she said again, "Pull up your zipper."

"Okay, Mommy."

After several more times, I was crying to Mom, "It's hot in here." She said, "*Not* that zipper."

Now, back to my first stint in college at SCSC. I did join the wrestling team. What a bunch of nuts on this team. There was one guy whose normal weight was like 150 lbs., who sucked down to about 125 lbs. The doctors told him he would be at a 0 percent body fat when he got to 123 lbs. (I think anything below 5 percent is actually unhealthy, but he went all the way down to 118 lbs. and was fairly successful.) He may have died since then, I don't know, but this was my first chink in the armor as far as my faith in doctors go. Basically, I stayed with the team for about a month or so. I actually wrestled once at the junior varsity level and won. I pinned some guy from the Coast Guard Academy with a headlock. I ended my college career undefeated and untied. I had a falling out with the head coach over Christmas break when the coach decided that the kids who live far away can live in a dorm over Christmas break. The guys who live close can drive to the school for the practices. I was in the middle. I did live nearly an hour away from campus, so I asked him to let me spend at least some time in the dorm so I wouldn't have to drive back and forth so many times. He said no, so I quit… I admit I wasn't too thrilled about the program at SCSC to begin with.

Even without wrestling anymore, there was plenty to do. I had numerous PE classes. Not to mention the running and weight lifting I have always done on my own. I admit that I went through college looking good, feeling good, and working hard at keeping in shape. Even though I was not on an organized team for the first time in nearly five years, I still had to keep in shape for the summers and the spring breaks when I would always go down to Daytona Beach or Fort Lauderdale. I did work out nearly every day, I still got my share of partying as well. SCSC was a great school for partying, and since the drinking age at that time was eighteen years old, there were numerous bars on or near campus, and every bar had their own particular night for cheap drinks. If you planned carefully, you could get drunk. Seven days a week, you can get a lot of value for your drinking dollar. And being a PE major, the workload was comfortable enough to accommodate this lifestyle. Although I partied, it was not seven days a week.

At one point, I got a job when I was a sophomore at SCSC. I began to coach wrestling as an assistant coach at Guilford High School. This was fun stuff. I did not make a lot of money for this, on the order of $500 a season (that would be three months), which comes to around or slightly less than a dollar an hour. But hey, I never said I would be rich. I just said that someday, I would have a heart attack. Since I was no longer participating on an organized team, I could coach one. This would complement my running program and would help to maintain my already-high level of fitness. If you have never wrestled, you will never know how hard it really is to go full steam for six minutes using every muscle in your body, suffice it to say it will keep you in great shape. The experience even turned out to be more rewarding than I expected. And over the next four years, I had a chance to watch these little immature squirts (that at times were hard to bear) grow up into big immature squirts. Several of them turned into semimature young adults who were not too hard to bear. It was a very unique and humbling experience, watching them grow. And I kept up my wrestling skills as well. One of the kids (a kid who was about my weight), who I had wrestled quite a bit over the four years, ended up as a state champ during his senior year. It was very rewarding for me to see him accomplish this.

There was one point when we were preparing for the state open, when we would practice with other schools. We would practice with other schools because only a couple of people from each team would qualify for the state open, and unless you got together with other schools, you may have a practice with only two or three kids—which could get very boring very fast, we felt strongly that you want to reward the kids for working hard all season long, not bore them to death. We happened to go to a school that had a heavyweight that was defending his state title. His record was 31–0. He weighed about 210 lbs. Of course, no one who was at this practice could handle him, so I was volunteered by the head coach, who insisted I wrestle him. I must have pinned him five or six times in the six minutes we wrestled. I really thought coaching improved my wrestling skills. But I knew in the back of my mind that wrestling was not a sport you can participate in for your whole life unless you were going to coach.

After coaching wrestling one year, the football coach approached me and told me that he liked the way I dealt with the kids and talked me into being the freshman football coach. I knew that my roommate from college who majored in recreation would be a perfect assistant coach. If you thought PE was easy, recreation made PE look like Einstein's theory of relativity; recreation majors actually had a course called basket weaving. This friend who was a recreation major needed a job, so I made him an assistant coach. He and I had a great time coaching football. We could take the full wrath of all the pain and frustration we had as high school players and take it out ten times worse on our team. I recall during our first day of practice, we had a freshman who was built like a brick shit house. He was about six feet tall, weighed 200 lbs., and most of this was muscle. We were doing a running drill with no pads on, just a light workout. When this kid (whose name I have forgotten) stopped, his legs buckled under him. We tried to get him to stand up, but it was too painful, so we let him stay on the ground for ten or fifteen minutes. We tried to get him up again, but we couldn't due to his pain. We decided to call an ambulance. After several minutes of observation, they took him away. We found out the next day that he actually broke both legs just below the knee. He almost died a couple of times due to blood clots that eventually formed. The doctor said that he was too developed muscularly for his body at that age, and basically, his bone growth did not keep up with his muscle growth, so when he stopped suddenly, his muscles actually helped to break his bones. This was a very sobering event indeed. My friend and I coached football on the freshman level for two years and were very successful, not because of raw talent but because our kids were very tough. We had so many tough drills that it turned them into little monsters. I think both teams ended up with a 5–2 record, which was far better than any varsity record was up until that point.

These freshmen football players were like the "bad news bears." I remember a game that we had with one of our archrivals. There was about thirty seconds left when we had the ball in a very close game. We were close to the opponents' goal line with no time-outs left. The clock was ticking. All of a sudden, the referee calls time-out. One of our kids was hurt, and it was the quarterback. We were quite upset. We got to our kid and looked at him; he was holding his balls. I asked him where it hurt. He said (making sure the ref wasn't listening), "Time was running out, so I made believe that I hurt my balls so I could stop the clock."

It was all we could do not to laugh. The high school rules said that if an injury time-out is called, the child that the time-out is called for must sit out of the game for at least one play, so we still lost the game. After two years of football coaching, we decided we had enough. There was a lot of time and much sacrifice that was necessary to coach football. The demands were too great. Along with our schoolwork, we were expected to coach, scout, and attend numerous meetings at odd hours. So sadly, we had to resign.

It was in my senior year when I got real serious about running. By this point, I weighed about 190 to 200 lbs. and was a fairly well built guy but really not built for running. If someone wants to see the picture of the ideal runner, get ahold of a Bill Rogers's picture. He is built like a walking lung. A good puff of wind would blow him over. It was in the late fall of 1978 that I decided that I wanted to run the Boston Marathon. I was twenty-two years old at the time, and as I have said, I was not built for running. I could not run real fast, but I was in good enough shape to run for a long period of time. I decided to run the Boston Marathon which traditionally was on the third Monday in April, Patriots' Day in 1979, my senior year. I knew the captain of the SCSC football team and told him what I was going to do. He thought it was as good an idea as I did. This guy was built like me; he was about six one and weighed about 200 lbs. He was a real tough kid. For instance, I remember running a couple of times with him in the streets of New Haven, which at times have some cars on them. I remember a car following us slowly, waiting to pass us, and he beeped his horn at us, probably because my friend was too far out into the street as he ran. He sniffed and snorted and worked up a huge hawker and promptly deposited it on the windshield of the previously mentioned car. The guy in the car just continued driving along. In this day and age, you must be more careful because if you do this to the wrong guy, you could get shot, or even seriously killed (ha-ha).

I was a guy who, in college, stayed in good shape. I would say that even though I exercised a lot, I did my share of goofing around as well. I drank, occasionally smoked pot, hash, but nothing to excess; you almost had to do this stuff just to exist at school. It was expected. I say this because when I mentioned my friend earlier, he was the only one I knew who did none of this. It was funny how he hung around with me and my roommates and managed to survive without any hanky-panky at all—no drinking, no smoking, no nothing. This friend was as straight as an arrow, nose-to-the-grindstone kind of guy. The only time I ever saw him drink anything was in Fort Lauderdale on spring break (I think I understand why he didn't drink after this evening.) We never seemed to have a lot of money, so one night we were all hungry (really hungry), so we decided to go to an all-you-can-eat-and-drink buffet for $5 or $6. We found out that you could only drink for one hour; this would keep people like us from staying all night to drink for free. This night I saw him drink his first beer (this after knowing him for a couple of years). Trust me, I think he was drunk on one beer, but he had several others as well. As alluded to earlier, you can imagine he liked to spit, so he got more and more unruly as the night went along. And the most vivid memory I recall from the whole spring break was leaving the restaurant, looking back at our table, and watching our last pitcher of beer filled to the brim with beer and slime (a good snotty hawker) hanging down from the pouring spout on the pitcher, almost down to the table. I practically threw up.

He and I made this commitment to run the Boston Marathon. And run we did. We used to run, not always together, depending on how our schedules were. But we would be running sixty to seventy miles a week. Usually, seven to ten miles a day during the week and on weekends, we would run one real light day, two to four miles on one day, and up to twenty miles on the hard weekend day. We did this schedule from approximately December of 1978 through the second week of April 1979. We trained in rain, snow, heat, and cold. We ran up and down some very big hills (after running ten to twelve miles, believe me, it actually gets easier to run up and down some hills rather than just running on a flat surface). I remember that on weekends for our long run, he and I would always try to run together. One Saturday, we couldn't get together to run. But I remember telling Scott my running mate and friend (who at times worked a security job for the school), "After work, wake me up, and we will run." I went to bed only to have him tickling my feet at three thirty in the morning, where we took off and ran about twenty miles.

We finished with the sun brightly shining at about 7:00 a.m., what a run.

If Boston was going to be hot we knew it would be a tough run for us since we both feared the heat. We were not built for running but we wanted to get some heat training. We went to Fort Lauderdale for spring break to do this. We tried to get some heat training, but we were not too crazy, so we decided to do our running at 5:00 or 6:00 a.m. every day of spring break. This way, we would not be running during the hottest part of the day, and this schedule would be the least disruptive in that most of the socializing on these breaks takes place in the afternoons and evenings. We also found that after a two-hour run, we could sneak a few extra hours of sleep if our six roommates were still sleeping. The room was crowded because we knew, the more people per room, the less it costs—no matter how uncomfortable it was. As it turned out, this was a mistake. This whole vacation was tough. We would go to bed at 1:00 to 3:00 a.m., wake up at 5:00 a.m., run two hours, and try to sneak a nap or two during the day, while we watched our roommates sleep, pick up girls, and get a lot of sleep. We thought that after the marathon was over, all this sacrifice would be worth it. We survived this vacation and went through our training until the second week in April. We talked to a few self-proclaimed experts on what we should do for the last week of our training. Their advice was that we should take it easy. Run only a couple of miles a day, if even that much, and we should feel real good during the marathon. We took this advice and just prayed all week that it would be a cool day for the marathon. That weekend, we drove up to my brother Jaime's place. Jaime was attending Boston College and was in a very convenient spot to launch our marathon attempt. Jaime, being an avid partier, and I were just hoping that when Monday morning came, he would be in good-enough shape to drive me and my friend to Hopkinton, Massachusetts, where the race starts. Our prayers were answered when we woke up that morning; the weather forecast was for a cloudy cool day with occasional drizzle, high near forty. We knew at this point we would probably succeed. Jaime dropped us off at Hopkinton and said he would be there at the finish line to pick us up after the race was over (or more appropriately, when we were finished running). We started the race at noon. There were about ten thousand people running in this thing. We were not registered runners, so we just lined up in the back and started. It took us about fifteen minutes to slowly work up from stutter steps and finally a real slow jog by the time we got to the start line. The eventual winner, Bill Rogers, was three and one-fourth miles into the race by the time we just started. The next twelve miles were fairly uneventful, and by taking a very light week of running before this event, we felt really good. It was around mile 14 when we found out that the race was officially over. Bill Rogers, as expected, did win. But we trudged on. As we went on mile 18–20, Scott got a little tired but kept on going. I was psyched at this point; we had reached "heartbreak hill," and it wasn't too bad. We were passing Boston College by now. I was trying to see my brother, who I later found out had a keg on the street with his friends as they watched the race. This is where some small problems crept up. We had never run this course before, so we had to rely on other people to tell us how far it was to the finish line. I would hear, "Only six miles to go," run for what seemed to be ten to fifteen minutes, then heard, "Only five and a half miles to go." It should have been four miles. This went on for what seemed like forever. It was frustrating for me, and it was really pissing off my friend, who was getting very tired by now. With about two to three miles left, I felt good, and he told me to go ahead, so I did. Once in Boston itself, I was not prepared for the number of turns I had to make before the end of the race. I envisioned maybe one or two turns, and I would see the banner. But it must have been seven or eight turns. After every turn, I expected to see the finish line and was getting increasingly disappointed when it wasn't there. Finally, I rounded that final elusive corner and saw the finish line about two hundred yards away. I sprinted and was almost drawn to tears. I was so elated by what I had done. I received this tin foil blanket and needed it because it got very cold very quickly after I stopped. My time was three hours and thirty minutes and forty-three seconds, and a marathon run is 26.2 miles. All I had to do now was wait for my friend. He came within five to ten minutes and was as happy as I was to complete this feat. Now one task left: to find my brother Jaime. Where was he?

At this point, I thought the hard part was over. I was with my buddy now, trying to find my brother. We both had our tin foil blankets on, and with the temperature hovering around forty degrees, I was cold. Scott was even colder; he was freezing and shaking. Maybe it was my fault for not planning for the ten gazillion people that were all hanging around the finish line. Maybe it was my brother's fault for partying a little too much and too long (I suspect the latter because he also put a few small pings in my car from some fender benders he admitted to having on the way to pick us up). The bottom line is that Scott and I were cold, tired, and trying to get back to Boston College. We sure did not feel like running or walking back to campus. I saw a guy who had just finished running, and he was wearing a BC sweatshirt. He was lucky enough to find his ride back to BC. We asked them to give us a lift; they gladly did. We arrived back on the BC campus to see all my brother's friends, but my car and brother were still missing. We took our nice warm showers, and my brother eventually showed up.

We had only one more obstacle to complete our mission. We had to get back to SCSC by Tuesday morning because I had a test at 10:30 a.m. that I couldn't get out of. As I mentioned, it was cool and drizzly (that helped us finish the marathon), but I found out that my windshield wipers did not work when I started to drive to SCSC. After about fifteen minutes, Scott was sleeping. And I had more than three hours of driving ahead of me. I was lucky to find a snow brush that had a rubber end that I could at least clean my windshield enough to see out of. With the drizzle, I could go maybe three or four minutes without cleaning the window, then I would have to roll the window down and stick this brush out the window, freeze my hand, and wipe the windshield off. The drizzle varied in intensity all the way back. Sometimes I could go ten or fifteen minutes at a clip, but if a truck or car passed me, I would have to clean off the windshield immediately. I was one very happy, yet very tired, camper when I finally got back to my dorm. I again went through this challenge with no physical problems. How did I know that I (we) dodged another bullet? I thought again what does not kill you would make you stronger.

I don't want to get ahead of myself, but I would regret not giving you a brief account of whatever happened to Scott. He, eventually, during his senior year at SCSC, applied to and obtained an assistant coaching job at Bowling Green University in Kentucky. He worked there for a couple of years. He also kept up his running. He ran in at least one or two more marathons. As I recall, he was training for the Boston Marathon in the spring of 1981. I did not keep in touch with him too often once I went on to OU (Oklahoma University). I got a call from my mother when I was a freshman at OU, who informed me that Scott had died. I heard my mother say something about a heart attack, but it was all a blur. I assumed he was running and just dropped dead. The next morning, I called his parents to give my condolences. Some guy answered the phone and said that his family was not taking any calls.

He said, "Who is this?"

I said, "Joe Mauro."

He said, "Joe who?"

And as soon as I said that, I heard Scott's mother in the background, "Joe Mauro? Joe Mauro? I want to talk to him."

We had only met a couple of times before. And she had always been a very nice, gracious woman. We had a good discussion (it was very sad I was so far from home I had no way of going to the funeral). She told me that he was training for the Boston Marathon. I said one was enough for me. He was just taking a nice, leisurely walk around a lake near where he lived and had a massive heart attack. That was scary. Here is a kid who played sports all his life. Unlike me, he never smoked, drank, or took drugs, and he just dropped dead. You know that with all the sports that he played, he must have seen numerous doctors every year, and no one ever found anything wrong or unusual.

This sort of thing is not as rare as one thinks. I would refer you to the stories about basketball player Hank Gathers and that famous runner Jim Fixx; both of whom died of massive heart attacks. It is possible we should drop theories about cholesterol, fat, high blood pressure, etc., and just say that each heart is born with a certain number of beats. When that number comes up, you are dead. Athletes actually die off sooner because they work out so often that they use up all their beats more quickly than, say, a couch potato. Sitting in front of a TV on the couch, eating a bag of pork rinds, your pulse is probably seventy. Running, your pulse is 130–150. Who will die quicker? Logic might now favor the athlete. I guess when your number is up, your number is up.

After the marathon in 1979, I had to try to top this for 1980. And I sure didn't want to do another marathon, so I decided to run every day in 1980. My goal was to run an average of five miles a day, six days a week, assuming I would take Sundays off. The only reason I mentioned this is to show what kind of a fanatic I was when it came to exercising. I would always do something, no matter how hard it was, simply to keep in shape. I would often do too much, though I never really injured myself running or lifting. I lived life on the edge of doing too much without knowing it.

CHAPTER 4

The College Years Round 2

Well, finally, I get to go to OU (Oklahoma University). After my graduation from SCSC, I applied to and got accepted to OU for meteorology. I was to begin in the fall semester of 1980. I remember telling my now-wife, then-girlfriend, about the acceptance. She did not seem too pleased. But I had to move on. I will not go into much detail about my love life down there but it was great because I am still married to this girl, even though we were not married or even engaged yet.

I remember the first time that I had to attend OU, I tried to leave at the last minute, which meant the morning before classes started. I arrived on the day classes actually started and talked to my adviser, the chairman of the meteorology department, a real hard-ass who for some reason liked me after a couple of meetings. I recall not knowing what or how long I had to remain in Oklahoma because I already had a four-year degree. But, I found out that I was in for another four-year stint in college because Oklahoma did not accept many credits from SCSC. I even had to repeat political science. In one sense, however, the fact that I had to repeat many classes helped me out. I knew most of the answers already. You see, the meteorology department was considered very hard and theoretical, and I bet that more than half of the kids who enter the program eventually quit.

There was a graduate course that to most of us would sound like one of the top 10 most fun courses based on its name: Severe Cumulous Convection, the study of severe thunderstorms. Would you believe that after two weeks, the course was canceled because all the graduate students quit. It was nothing but differential equations and mathematical theory, too hard even for the smartest in the school.

I had a big advantage over all the other undergraduates: I didn't care about any of my grades, except for those in meteorology. I had a roommate that was one year ahead of me. This kid tried to impress everyone as to how hard meteorology was. He would often stay up all night. He wouldn't sleep two or three nights a week and just kept ragging about how hard the meteorology program was. I thought he was trying to impress everyone, but as it turned out, he was just dumb. He eventually dropped out. As I matriculated through those four years, my conception of the program was that it was hard but not that bad. I had an average of two meteorology classes as well as a math course every semester. Without caring about US history, political science, biology, gym, it was a very manageable load.

The teachers there were all characters as well. They would go through incredible lengths to irritate the shit out of you in class. Outside of class, they were really nice people. We used to have parties with them, the Christmas party, Groundhog Day party, etc. These guys were experts on not mixing business with pleasure. One professor used to get stoned with us and go to our regular Friday night shot parties. During classes, he was a real pain in the ass.

I maintained keeping in shape in Oklahoma. That was some real heat training. It is a hot place, especially in the late spring through early fall. I used to run with the professors at lunchtime. They would all gather around and run a couple of miles with each other and a few chosen students. I also would run on my own, so I was probably still averaging about five miles at least five or six days a week. I also managed to do what I call golf a couple of times a week.

After a couple of months, I hooked up with a few other people from the northeast that I found there. We had our own little club. We would go out and party, as well as lift weights and run. Another thing I got addicted to, along with my new friends, was softball. I recall that during my last two years in Oklahoma, I was in three separate leagues, and on weekends, we would always find some corner of the state to play in a tournament. We were playing 225 to 250 games a year—this while maintaining a 3.5+ GPA in meteorology. My GPA in other areas was falling apart, but who cared, that was just a way that OU forced my father to pay more for me by taking classes I had already taken. There should be a law against this.

That has always been a pet peeve with me that these colleges have the gall to constantly raise tuitions and charge you outrageous prices for books and parking permits even though half the time, you couldn't find a place to park on campus. Basically, any college will extract every penny you have, extract your parents for every penny they have, yet be the first to beg you for donations after you graduate and have a job they didn't help you get. They charge outrageous prices on any souvenirs that actually advertise their school, an OU shirt will cost you $20, and you are advertising their school. They should give this stuff away to OU students. I have the same feeling about places like Disney World. When you go there, spend hundreds or thousands of dollars to get there, then spend money on their hotels to stay there, then spend hundreds of dollars to attend their parks, literally spending thousands of hard-earned dollars to patronize their business—they charge exorbitant-rates for souvenirs. A small Mickey Mouse doll will cost you $40 when it costs a quarter to make (most likely by breaking some child labor law in Taiwan or China). If you spend all this money to visit Disney World, why can't they give you a few Mickey Mouse dolls as a PR program? Sell to the people who don't patronize you, not the people that do. Sorry for this aside, but things like this bother me—a poor guy struggling for his family to gather enough money for a little fun and a multibillion dollar business trying to bleed him for everything he's got. Try to get a McDonald's hamburger in Disney World, and you would eventually go broke feeding a family of four on fast food. Okay, where was I? That's right, I was in Oklahoma, running, lifting weights, playing too much softball. I know what you are thinking: softball is for beer-drinking fat people who can't play baseball. Wrong. Play five or six games a day, like we did in many tournaments, you will be stiff and trying to avoid playing the next day, even though often we had to.

We know I am exercising a lot with no adverse effects, but the clock is ticking. So how is my social life going? After I lived in a dorm at OU for a year, I decided that it was too noisy, and with no real privacy, so I decided to room with a senior, off campus. By my sophomore year, the first summer after my freshman year, I managed to get engaged to my lovely soon-ex-wife-to-be, Sue, as mentioned before we are still married.

In 1981, we went on a windjammer cruise off the Maine coast toward the end of the summer, and one thing led to another, and I said, "Why don't you quit your job and move to Oklahoma with me, and just live together?"

That went over fine with Sue, but her father, a superior court judge, had something to say about it. I remember going to Sue's house one evening to discuss this with her father, and as I drove toward her street, she was running to my car, saying, "Don't go in there, he will kill you, he will not let us live together."

I realized that he did have a very strong argument after we talked about it in-depth.

He said, "It's just not done."

I said, "It's done every day."

"No, it's just not done."

"But we are not kids." (I was twenty-four; she was twenty-two.) "We can do this and make it work."

He said—you guessed it—"It's just not done."

I guess if you just say "it's just not done" enough, you can't argue that anymore, so we kind of agreed to get married the following winter at Christmas break on January 2, 1982. By the way, since that time, "it's just not done," has occurred twice with Sue's siblings.

After Sue and I got married, we lived with my roommate for one semester before we got our own apartment the following summer. While we were living with him, a funny incident occurred one night. He had a date with this girl that we both knew from the meteorology department. I should tell you that my favorite alcoholic beverage at that time was Drambuie. I didn't drink this too much, but enough to have an empty bottle or two hanging around the apartment. I also, from time to time, ate bacon for breakfast. This could have been a contributing factor toward having my heart attack.

I would pour the bacon grease in one of my old Drambuie bottles because we know, we can't pour this grease down the drain; it would just clog up (much like it would clog up a major artery). I had this bottle about half full of bacon grease at the time. My roommate woke up one morning and told me about his date. He and his girlfriend both got sick and threw up a couple of times. He said that he thought my Drambuie was bad.

I said, "Good, you shouldn't steal someone else's Drambuie in the first place."

He said when he mixed it with chocolate milk, it seemed to curdle. Who in their right mind would mix great liquor like Drambuie with chocolate milk? Even real Drambuie might curdle with chocolate milk. Needless to say, the girl, my new wife, and the whole meteorology department thought he was a twit after this. I didn't miss moving out on him that summer.

While I was going to OU, I would be remiss if I didn't mention my part-time job at the National Severe Storms Lab (NSSL). I made $6 or $7 an hour doing what most OU students would pay to do. I worked for the NSSL for three years. This was a cool place. As you probably have heard, Oklahoma is in tornado alley. Most of the meteorology students, being poor but interested as hell in weather (if you were willing to go through these classes to get a degree in meteorology, you better be at least moderately interested in weather), would cram into a car. Of course, the more people you got to go with you, the cheaper it was per person. More people can chip in for gas to go chase tornadoes. It was very interesting. But after I learned that I could get paid for doing this, my decision was easy. I would rather chase tornados with NSSL than get all cramped up in an OU student's car to chase them. NSSL would study thunderstorms for nine months a year. But for three months a year, they would chase severe thunderstorms and tornadoes. This way, they would accumulate data to study for the next several years, using the data to verify their very new Doppler radar. The story I heard is that it was almost by accident when they discovered what a TVS, tornado vortex signature, looked like on Doppler. They saw a glitch on the radar, and some chasers who documented everything realized the glitch coincided with the tornado and the time it was reported on the ground. I chased tornadoes for my first year with the OU chase team, before I got smart and worked for NSSL and got paid to drive for them. My wife used to get calls like, "I may not be home tonight," "I may be in Kansas or Texas or whatever." This was a really unique experience that I enjoyed a lot. There are a lot of stories to tell about chasing, but this book is not about that; it is about Joe's heart attack. Perhaps the stress from this contributed to the heart attack.

While I was in Oklahoma, we did get some extra exercise twice a year. We used to "punch doggies." My wife and I and several friends from OU got together with one of the girls (an Oklahoman we knew) and whose father was a county judge in Oklahoma and a cattle rancher. He owned two hundred to three hundred cows and bulls. Twice a year, we would go to his farm in Paul's Valley, Oklahoma, early in the morning to perform this task. The rules were that he would supply all the food you could eat, all the tobacco you could chew, and all the beer you could drink. We would do some strange things with these cows and bulls—including cutting their balls off, dehorning them, giving them shots, having a vet give them pregnancy tests, weighing them, and being ankle-deep in cow dung. Back then, my wife was skinny, five feet tall, and no more than 100 lbs. soaking wet (that is what you get from standing behind a cow). She would stand in a stall with about fifty cows in it. These cows would be so scared of her they would all turn away from her and hide in the corner of the pen. They thought that if they couldn't see her, she couldn't see them. We slept very well on the nights we "punched doggies." This girl's father, whom we called Pops, took care of us. I don't know if he liked us because his daughter liked us, or he really appreciated us helping with his cows. But he was an avid OU football fan. Back then, OU did play some good football. I think they even won a national championship in one of the years I attended OU. When there was a home game, we would all meet at one of the local bars at about 10:00 a.m. The games usually started at noon or 1:00 p.m., so this would provide us with plenty of time to drink. Pops would usually have all of us on a tab before the game. We would drink until drunk, then we would go to the game then hook up after the game and usually go out and chow down. Students like us had very limited budgets, so these binge's every other week or so in the fall really helped. One of these days, I may just go down to see him and punch doggies with my kids. I regret having lost touch with him.

CHAPTER 5

After Eight Years Finally Out of College

After I graduated OU, I got a job in Austin, Texas, in June of 1984. The company's name was the Texas Weather Service. The owner was hush-hush because he did not want the folks where he worked to know that he was doing this on the side. Austin is a nice town, but it was a hot place, and I must say again, I don't enjoy heat. The Texas Weather Service worked out of a TV station in Austin. Somehow he managed to lease some space from this TV station. The deal was that the main weatherman could consult with me (a guy with a meteorology degree), about weather, because he really did not know too much about weather. For that, we would get a workspace and access to the weather data we needed. The first day I was in Texas, I thought it would be a very short stay. We had to argue our way into the TV station; they didn't want any part of us. But finally, we talked our way in.

The arranged deal was that I would work six days a week. He would work only one day a week. The owner had another job, so I guess I understood. He also gave me a beeper so that he could always contact me, although one thing about me is that I hate phones and beepers. But beepers are worse! No matter what you are doing, you have to drop it and call whoever beeped you. I worked six days a week and Sunday, my day off, he would beep at me at least eight to ten times. I wasn't making much money doing this job. As it turned out, I was working seven days a week, counting the time I was beeped all day long on Sundays.

Working out in Texas was a little different than I was used to. I could not find a convenient weight room, so my main exercise was running. I would run and play in one softball league. Still, I maintained a good level of fitness.

Christmas was approaching, and I realized that I really did not like the job, or Austin, for that matter. I have always lived in the northeastern United States. We have four seasons, and I feel that something was wrong with a place where sweat would be dripping off your brow when you were doing your Christmas shopping. December was here, and my boss decided to call an executive meeting of the board of directors of the Texas Weather Service (that would be me and him). He regretted to inform me that with only one client, and his inability to get more clients, he was going to fold up shop around mid-December. I acted sad, but that was the best news I had heard in years. I was going to go home and be there before Christmas. I have not mentioned it enough, but let me make it clear that my wife has been a good sport throughout all my moves. She found new jobs everywhere we went and did no complaining about it. I think she was happy that we were heading back to New England but I don't think as happy as me.

CHAPTER 6

Back in Connecticut

We were finally homeward bound in December 1984. This was going to be great. I have no job, but I am sure I could live at home until I get my feet on the ground. At this time, I really didn't know what was going on jobwise. I know jobs for meteorologists were rare, indeed; I knew jobs like metallurgists were common. I thought, since they were spelled so closely, the job description would be similar. That couldn't be further from the truth. I applied for many jobs out of my field just to do something, but nobody wanted me. I remember I wanted to work for the maintenance department in Branford, Connecticut. I sent a résumé to the maintenance director and followed it up with an interview. The guy practically laughed at me.

He said, "You have gone to college for eight years, have a degree in meteorology, what do you want to work in the maintenance department for?" He just said you are overqualified. "I'll call you after the interview process is over." I never heard from him again.

In between all the résumés I was sending out and interviews I had, I was running and lifting weights, and now I was doing sit-ups and push-ups as well, but the job thing was becoming a dead end. My wife had no trouble getting a job in some tomato canning factory in North Haven, Connecticut. I have to admit that I felt a little guilty. Sue was working. I was home for the most part, sitting around in my pajamas, doing nothing but a little running and lifting; I was doing nothing—watching TV and eating three squares a day that my parents were supplying. I wish I could do that forever.

My dad would always get on my case about getting a job. He would say, "You have to network, talk to people, send out hundreds of cover letters and résumés." He said, "Nothing ever happens when you are sitting at home, doing nothing. You have to pound the pavement."

My father still believes there are thousands of jobs in meteorology all over the place. I sent out some résumés for meteorology, but it really is a limited field—especially when you only have a bachelor of science degree. If you had a master's or a doctorate degree, you could get into research jobs, which are probably more common. With all the air pollution and water pollution, global warming, there are many hot topics to research.

I did not and still do not want to pursue a master's or PHD degree in meteorology. I can't be a student forever. I think eight years of college is enough for anybody. I did have one interview in Boston for some kind of air pollution research job. I don't know how I even got the interview. I guess they liked my résumé even though I only had a bachelor of science degree. This was my first real interview since the maintenance department in Branford, for which I was overqualified. But for this one, I was very underqualified. I remember driving from Madison, Connecticut (where I was living unemployed with Mom and Dad), to Boston at 5:00 a.m. for a 9:00 a.m. interview. It was about a three-hour ride, and I was a little concerned about getting caught in rush hour. The biggest memory I had from that day was my tight shoes—which I borrowed from my father like two sizes too small. Somehow, the closest I could park was about a mile away. By the time I arrived at the interview, my feet were dead. This is not a good way to start an interview. For me, this felt like strike 1 and 2.

I sat in the reception area for about fifteen minutes, and I was led into the interview room. I expected one guy to talk to me, when in fact there was a panel of five people throwing all kinds of weird questions about air pollution at me. I don't think I even got one question correct at this interview. I had no clue. I felt stupid, especially when I realized that this had absolutely nothing to do with weather—remember, that thing I was trained for? My only consolation is that deep inside, I knew they were wrong for calling me for the interview. Needless to say, I never heard from them again. All I had to do now was walk a mile back to my car with my blistered feet. It took two or three days to recover from that.

After a couple of months of doing absolutely nothing, I got a painting job for a local painting contractor. I was still hunting for a weather job. At this time, my chances seemed rather low for actually getting one. But I was making about $10 an hour, so I felt a little productive. My dad was still saying, "Network, you will never get a weather job painting, send out résumés talk to people, make phone calls, yadda, yadda, yadda."

I managed to save a little money along the way. Ten dollars an hour is not a lot of money, but expenses were low, I was living at home, I saved some money. There were many days when it would rain or things would be slow for one reason or another, and I would have some time off, where I could be found in my pj's watching TV. I would always get my workouts in, but I seemed to be getting no closer to my career goals. The end of my painting career came into view on one job I was doing. There was a contemporary house that the boss got. It had cathedral ceilings, and it was a huge house. I remember that the boss took me there one morning and left me there and said that we will be painting all the ceilings in the house, nothing but the ceilings, then he left. And for the next two weeks, I worked every day in that house. I think I only saw him once or twice in passing. He did nothing on that job; it was all me.

This boss, by the way, was so cheap he actually paid me off the books. I was a subcontractor. He paid me in cash, so he did not have to pay FICA, taxes, Social Security, insurance, or anything for me. It was my job to take it out of my $10 an hour. This killed me at tax time the following year, but I don't want to get into that at this point. I keep telling you these stories so you can see the pressures, anxieties, and stress I have endured up to this point to get, or to earn, a heart attack.

Back to the ceilings—after about two weeks of doing the ceilings in this house, I saw the bill that my boss gave the homeowners. I wasn't prying, but it was left on the kitchen table, open for the world to see. And that cheapskate of a boss billed these people $6,800 for the ceilings. I am not against the guy making a buck; he did get the job in the first place. But I figured that he paid me $10 an hour, forty hours a week for two weeks. That means he paid me $800 (remember, especially you, IRS agents, who are reading this book, even though he didn't do anything illegal, it was my stupidity as a subcontractor that gave him this right to take advantage of me). This guy had to pay for supplies. Let's say he spent $1,000 on supplies; that meant that he cleared at least $5,000 on this job alone with me doing all the work.

I told him I wanted $15 an hour, which I knew I deserved if I was making him this kind of money. I knew he could afford it. I found out he didn't wear the pants in the family; he wimped out and said, "I have to ask my wife." She did the books and said no to the $15 and said, "I can give you twelve." I said, "See ya later."

I don't like being taken advantage of. So I was unemployed again, but I had saved up enough money to give my wife a well-deserved vacation. I knew that her mother, who was working as a nurse for a public school in Cheshire, Connecticut, was going with the French club or some group on a trip to Germany, France, and a few of those countries; for approximately a thousand dollars, I could send Sue as well. I thought she and her mother would have a great time.

So for a Christmas present, I gave her some francs, lira, and rubles, and then I shocked her with these tickets for a plane trip to Europe.

In the meantime, I quit the painting job and started selling life insurance. This is a business that my father started in and was very successful at. I was not overly qualified for this; if you could breathe, they would hire you. Sounds easy, doesn't it? If you didn't sell, you would quickly get fired, or even more likely, quit, because you work on commission. You don't sell, you don't get paid.

I don't want to get into a long story here for a job I held for such a short time. But I was experiencing some success, and I could have seen me doing this job for a while, but another twist in the road presented itself. It was late March of 1986, and I had sent my wife to Europe on her European vacation. My parents, at the same time, were also out of town. They were in Rome on a work-related trip. So I was home alone for a week in late March. You can guess what I did. I performed my favorite activity. I called in sick for a couple of days and stayed home in my pj's and watched TV. At this point, I didn't even send out résumés or anything. I figured I would sell insurance and never get a weather job. After all, I had been home for almost a year and a half with no luck. Perhaps my father was right. Although I would never admit it and as it turned out, I never had to. As I was sitting home watching TV one day, the following sequence of events occurred:

While I was watching TV, the phone rang. It was MasterCard.

"Do you want a credit card with a ten thousand dollar limit?"

I said, "I don't really have a job."

She said, "Is your name Joe Mauro."

I said, "Yes, but you probably want my father, he has a job."

She said that if my name was Joe Mauro, I could have a credit card. So, I got one. Then I got a call from the National Weather Service in Raleigh Durham, North Carolina, and they informed me that I could have a job as a meteorologist in North Carolina. With

Sue in Europe and my parents in Rome, I told him to give me a couple of days to decide. Then I got a call from some guy named Frank from some weather service I never heard of. I asked him how he got ahold of my résumé; he said that another local weather service had sent him the résumé. I made an arrangement to have an interview, and I finally got a job in the area I was trained for, a real weather company. I started on April 16, 1986. At first, I had reservations about the job due to the fact that I would have to take a pay cut (from selling insurance), but once I saw the weather maps again, I just had to get a job in weather. Is that the end of my story? No! Sorry. But we are getting closer to the interesting part.

CHAPTER 7

My Family

Now that I had a job, and I had been married for four years already, it was time to nest and start a family. It is not as easy as it sounds. After the first year, I finally became a homeowner. My wife and I bought our first (and only) house in Ansonia, Connecticut, about fifty miles away from Westchester County Airport where I worked. The reason I live so far from work is that with the limited income I was making, I couldn't afford to live any closer. But at least, for the time being, it didn't matter. What did hurt my master plan, however, was my luck. Since I was born, my luck with things like this has always sucked. Real estate values have gone up since the beginning of time; even my real estate agent said home values would never go down. Of course, that was true, until I bought a house. Five to ten years ago, I tried to sell it a couple of times to move closer to work, but I would lose about $20,000 to do so. Now I can't, because the kids are in school, they have friends, and I don't want to move them and upset everything.

By the way, this house, though far from work, is in a very nice area where I could run on some fairly dead roads. We live on top of a hill in a very quiet neighborhood. The only bad thing is that by living on top of a hill, you always start your runs downhill (which makes it easy to warm up) but you always end up your runs by running

53

up hill—which kills you and evidently causes heart attacks, ergo the name of this book. We also have a YMCA located just eight-tenths of a mile away from our house, so now I run and lift weights on a regular basis.

On August 15, 1989, we had our first child. We named him Christopher Joseph Mauro (CJM), which happens to be the name of the bar where I picked up my wife. This kid was a blessing from day 1—it was a great experience having him. As luck would have it, my wife had a difficult time with the birth, getting all kinds of false labor pains and the like. We spent about three days in the hospital during the end of her pregnancy, waiting and waiting and waiting and waiting. The doctors would say, "Let's wait and see what, if anything, will happen."

After three days straight, I told Sue I can't use up all my sick days doing nothing, so I have to go to work. So I went to work. I just set foot in the office when the phone rang. It was Sue. She said they are doing a caesarian section. I left immediately, went to the hospital where I missed the birth of my son by about one minute. But I saw him come out of the operating room right after I arrived at the hospital. I was thirty-two years old with a brand-new son. Now, instead of exercising to just keep in shape, I had to exercise so that as my son grew up, I could keep up with him.

On May 18, 1993, I was blessed with my second child, Tracey Mauro. My wife was having more problems late in the pregnancy with Tracey. This time, along with the false labor pains, my wife swelled up quite a bit; she kind of looked like an engorged tick. Her ankles were almost the size of my thighs. So the last several days, she was once again in the hospital. Is this sounding familiar yet? This time, I took maybe one sick day and figured that the baby was three or four days away, these doctors did what they do best, just wait and see what happens next. But when I got into work, I got a call. Again, the second I arrived at the hospital, they are doing another C-section.

This time, I arrived before the baby came. I saw Sue's mother in the room. She was dressed in a blue nurse's uniform, waiting to see the C-section.

As soon as I got to the room, she said, "Tell the nurse you are here, and you can go in."

But as soon as she said this, a nurse came in and said, "Let's go."

No time for me to get changed, so I missed another one by seconds.

I don't want to get into a long dialogue of how these kids were, but to any prospective parents out there, I must say having children is the best experience I have ever had. I would not give up this experience for anything on the planet. Let me also say that after having Chris, I thought the first three years of a child's life was not too hard on the parents; he was easy. After having Tracey, my mind was changed. She was a pain in the ass for the first three years of her life. I really wanted to put her back in. I must admit, after the first three years, both kids were fairly easy to get along with. But for my first three years with her, all I could think is that, with an average of 300,000,000 sperm, Tracey's sperm cell had to be the one that swam the fastest. She was lucky to make it to three years old.

Something rare happened after Tracey. Because we had two kids and my wife worked and I worked, it took a lot of time and coordination to get things done. There was about a one-year period I did not exercise at all. This was a strange experience for me. After a couple of months, I realized how good I felt because I didn't work out. I never noticed before how much my ankles, knees, back, and neck hurt while I was running, until I stopped and they felt better than I could ever remember. Because I always ran, I thought this stiffness and pain was normal, but when I stopped running and all of a sudden something was missing (pain and stiffness), I was amazed.

After a year off, I gained some weight, which I didn't mind so much. But I felt fat, and at that point, I figured that I liked to eat and if I am going to eat, I am going to run and exercise to work it off. So here I go again.

I must say that though I have never been a skinny guy, I have not been fat either. I am about six feet tall, large boned, and weigh between 200 and 220 lbs. for the most part. I don't like to see doctors much because my thought is that if you feel good, why go; they will probably find something wrong. I also think they are sometimes worse than weathermen when it comes to diagnosing things. I really have heard some war stories. Briefly there was a girl that goes to my kid's school, a first-grader. She had trouble walking for months, and the doctors kept saying she had Lyme disease. It turns out that after almost a year, they said she had cancer. She went through chemo and radiation for a little over a year. I don't want to say it caused my heart attack, but she lost her battle only a week or so before my heart attack. This is a truly sad story, but who knows what could have happened had this been diagnosed accurately at the beginning. They say the earlier you catch the cancer, the more curable it is. She lost a year.

CHAPTER 8

My General Health and the Building Pressure from My Job

As long as I can remember my blood pressure has always been borderline high (about 140/90) my cholesterol between 180 to 200, and my HDL (good cholesterol) always high from all the working out. I had a checkup in January or February 1997, and everything looked good, even on an extensive blood test.

As I went through the late 'nineties, I continued to run and lift weights at the YMCA until the disaster hit. As far as taking care of myself, I think I have done that. The only thing I left out was that I did, over the past several years, drink a glass of wine every night, which should also lessen my chances of having a heart attack.

Briefly let me describe the negatives, the things that have contributed to the heart attack, of which there are only a few. First is a family history, but only a few relatives had a problem with their hearts. My father had a heart attack when he was fifty-eight. He turned out fine, and he is now seventy years old. I had only a couple of great-uncles that had heart problems. Second, as I mentioned before, I always had borderline numbers as far as blood pressure and cholesterol go, good HDL levels, and a blood pressure borderline high. As stated, some numbers are borderline, but not sufficient to cause a heart attack at the age of forty-three! My eating habits were not bad, not great. I used to, from time to time, have sausages, suppressato, boneless barbecued spare ribs, etc., but that was one of the motivations for my heavy exercise—because I like to eat. I was never really obese. I would usually weigh between 200 lbs. to 220 lbs. for the most part. I did consume a lot of caffeine, not so much with coffee but in lots of Coke, probably averaging about a quart a day—which I admit is a little much (apparently, it was).

I guess another factor was stress. There are two types I suffer from. One is social stress (anxiety). I don't feel comfortable in many social situations and am often forced by my wife and family to do many things I prefer not to do—such as, dine in fine restaurants, go on vacation to faraway places. I never traveled well and, up until now, never thought this would kill me. It was just something I had to learn to deal with. It has always been hard for me to just relax doing nothing.

The other type of stress is job related. I am a type A personality when it comes to work. I like to come in and work hard and get my job done. The problem is that my job did not work that way. For example, painting houses, you start, work your ass off, and when you finish, you go home. At work in the weather office, there are certain things that must be done on a regular basis. There would be perhaps an hour or two of hard work. The rest of the eight-hour shift is taking care of last-minute Charlie's that forgot to tell you to do something before. Being in a service organization, the customer is always right, and we must accept their unreasonable requests even when at the last minute, these jerks remembered they were going to Denver in fifteen minutes. Now it was my problem to create a weather package that would safely and legally get them from Miami to Denver, avoiding any severe weather, etc., and send it to them (fifteen minutes ago). We had to do this with smiles on our faces. The aviation weather business is tough, but don't get me wrong. I love weather but have always hated phones and repeating myself, so what do you think 90 percent of my job was? You guessed it.

I forecast weather for corporate aircraft. Many Fortune 500 companies have their own little fleets of aircraft. And I must plan everything so these aircraft get around the world safely and expeditiously. Take for example, a pilot that wants to go from New York to San Francisco. Our company has the capability to do everything that aircraft and crew need to take this trip. We will give them safe and reliable weather forecasts; we will create and file their flight plans, sell them fuel, and take care of handling, overflight permits, limos, catering, and more. We make hotel arrangements for the crew and their passengers. Sometimes, I think, in dealing with corporate pilots, they are not as well trained as commercial pilots who fly for American Airlines or Southwest Airlines or some of the other big, commercial airlines.

I dealt with helicopter pilots, who insisted we hold their hands to get them through a trip. I had pilots who, having a trip ten hours from now, call every hour on the hour and half hour—and their copilots will call as well—about what the weather conditions are now and what is expected in ten hours, nine hours, eight hours, etc. Another thing that adds stress is people who take advantage of the system. For example, if you know an accountant, do you ask him for free income tax advice? If you go regularly to a deli, do you ask for free meat in your sandwich? If you know a doctor, do you ask for a free flu shot? Of course not, if you have any class at all. It would be considered very insulting to the beggee. It would be in bad taste to take advantage of any similar situation like this. So too, are poor manners with so many pilots you have to help professionally, getting sidetracked and being constantly interrupted by people looking for a few golf forecasts for next Saturday. These people should listen to the radio or use the Internet.

It is unfair to other clients who don't take advantage of this free-bie-type behavior. We have to accommodate these requests much of the time. When it is busy at work, it is very busy; when it is slow, it is slow, and we can kick back, relax, and enjoy the moment—because it probably won't last long. We have to cater to these pilots like we have to cater to spoiled children and tell them if it is going to rain on their picnic two weeks from next Thursday. Another thing, we have to answer many questions that we don't know the answer to. When you get as precise as we have to, you can rarely get a perfect forecast. We can't simply say it will be sunny or cloudy; we have to say the ceiling will be three hundred feet; the visibility will be three-fourths mile in fog and drizzle, and the wind will be 150 degrees at twelve knots. I don't think in sixteen years that I have ever hit a forecast exactly. Another thing that annoys me, especially when we are busy, something like this will happen, and this exact thing did happen to me (again, I won't mention any names until I retire).

We had a rule at work—which was rather stupid, but they pay me, so sometimes I even have to do stupid things.

When we put someone on hold, we can't say, "Weather Department, please hold."

We must say, "Weather Department, can you hold?"

We have to be polite. Most times, I say, "Weather Department, can you hold, thank you," without even waiting for a response and put them on hold immediately.

But I made a mistake one day. It was a really busy day. There were thunderstorms and even isolated reports of severe weather. I recall the phones ringing off the hook. I was briefing one pilot and quite literally trying to get him to navigate around intense thunderstorm activity, which is a big threat for aircraft. Another phone rang, and I said, "Weather Department, can you hold?"

The guy said no, so being a good meteorologist, the only thing I could guess is that he was in a plane and needed some quick timely weather information. So I put the original pilot on hold (the guy I interrupted in the first place) and got back to, let's call him, Captain Emergency, and said, "How can I help you?"

He said, "I am having an outdoor party on Saturday evening, is it going to rain?"

If this isn't taking advantage, I don't know what is, and we—the people in the company on the low end of the food chain—have to cater to these spoiled brats. Come to think of it, I just realized this behavior and the stress it created probably caused my heart attack. I guess I have little tolerance for inconsiderate moochers that do these things every day.

Here is another example of our company's incompetence. The president of our company was in town one busy day. We had about three or four incoming lines, two or three people answering the phone. Once in a while, we have to put people on hold for a brief period. On this day, we had two people working the phones and four phone lines ringing. The president heard us interrupting our weather briefings to put people on hold. So instead of saying we need more help to do the briefings, he suggested we needed more phone lines. Then we could interrupt even more briefings to put people on hold.

We also get a fair share of pilots who will call us up and put us on hold. Now, isn't that valuable time wasted? If you can't talk, don't make the call. Call later if you wish, but don't waste our time.

These are actual questions that I have had to entertain from some of the bozos I have had to deal with over the past sixteen years. Tell me I'm not dealing sometimes with inexperienced pilots. Yikes! People actually put their lives in the hands of these people. I just hope that there are not too many technical terms that would mask some of the stupidity I have to deal with every day. Please note this is just a sample of the thousands of questions I have heard. I have to apologize to my dad, because he always has said that there is no such thing as a stupid question. I think these will prove him wrong. Tell me there is no stress on my job.

This is my stupid question list:

1) Me: From here to Washington, it will be clear and 7+.
   Pilot: What kind of clear will it be? This is a helicopter.
2) Me: The wind is calm.
   Pilot: What direction is that from?
3) Pilot to me: Is that 20Z California time or 20Z New York Time?
   (It's all the same.)
4) Secretary: After three inches of snow has already fallen with six to nine inches more to fall, as well as an expected nasty mix of sleet and freezing rain, and they're not calling it a storm?
5) Pilot: What time will the snow start?
   Joe: Seven a.m. to 10:00 a.m.
   Pilot: Is that in the morning or the afternoon?
6) Horse racetrack… It is 1:00 p.m., and they say, "We have rain and thunder, I didn't know this was supposed to happen."
   I said, "Well, the forecast says chance for a shower or thunderstorm until 3:00 p.m."
   He said, "Oh, I don't read those things."
   Why do we give them a forecast?
7) Pilot gives me a weather request. I say, "Is this going to a fix base operator or hotel?"
   The pilot says, "No, it's going to a fax."
8) I ask a lady from a newspaper how to spell *Gail*. I said, "How do you spell her name?"
   The lady said, "G-a-l-e, and by the way, she is a man."
   Not stupid, just cute.

9) I say, "Yes, we will get four to six inches of snow on grass, two to three inches snow on roads."
Pilot: Is it going to stick?

10) 6/25/97 Joe talking to a pilot
Pilot: I am going from Roanoke to Dulles Airport.
Me: Okay, you have one intense thunderstorm about ten to fifteen miles NE of Roanoke, go anywhere you want, but don't go northeast to get out of Roanoke.
Pilot: How about if I head for Montigello (or something like that)?
Me: Fine, where is Montigello?
Pilot: Just northeast of here.
(Not the brightest bulb in the Christmas tree.)

11) This would be funny if it was not true.
It was a mostly cloudy day. A pilot called me and asked, "Will there be any rain today?"
I said, "Most likely, no."
The pilot said there was enough rain in Norwalk to wet the parking lot. We were all kind of surprised (especially since I just drove through Norwalk ten minutes ago to get to work). Anyway, he called back five minutes later and said he made a mistake; the parking lot was wet because someone was washing their car.

12) It's February. A pilot asks me what Montreal's temperature will be running the next couple of days. I say, "Low to midthirties."
He asks, "Is that Celsius or Fahrenheit?"
(I keep knocking, but nobody's answering.)

13) I asked a pilot what his itinerary was. He asked, "What is an itinerary?"

I could go on, but I don't want this book to be longer than war and peace. I hope you can see that it is really hard to soar with eagles when you are dealing with turkeys.

After reading these again, it's a wonder that I made it this long at my job. Aside from this stress that the job created, the only bad habit I had was chewing tobacco. I have done this for years, since I was about twenty years old. I thought that you could get cancer from that stuff, but I never thought for a second that it could cause heart problems. I know cigarettes cause a whole variety of heart and lung ailments, but I always thought, perhaps blindly, that it was the process of smoking that did most of the damage. But from what several nurses in the hospital said, nicotine is a stimulant that could raise blood pressure. That and the fact that I drank a large amount of Coke on a regular basis kept my heart very stimulated and my blood pressure high most of my waking hours. Even though I have quit the chewing of tobacco, I would like to one day find out my blood pressure, then chew tobacco, and find out what it is maybe fifteen to twenty minutes after I started chewing to see if there is a big difference. Seeing I had a heart attack, I should take volunteers (from the people who asked the stupid questions) so perhaps they could die, instead of me. Fortunately, up until now, I have had absolutely no health problems.

Up to this moment, you know everything about me, but then the shocker came: imagine all that exercise wasted. How many hours of sweating, running, lifting, pushing, and pulling weights did I do? Did it all go for naught with only one bad habit? No one can tell exactly what caused the thing to happen, especially with everyone afraid of frivolous lawsuits.

CHAPTER 9

Events Leading to My Heart Attack

It is time to review the heart attack and the events leading up to it. I guess the first sign of trouble was in September of 1999. I know that the company I work for financed a golf outing to be held be on September 23. On September 21, I had my first chest pains. I was lifting weights early in the morning (6:30–7:00 a.m.). When I was through lifting, I remember within the hour, I had a burning sensation in the middle of my chest. It wasn't a particularly painful thing, but I must say, there was discomfort. I sat down for half an hour or so before I had to leave for work, but it wasn't until I was driving to work that I noticed that the pain lessened. By noon or so, the pain was completely gone. At that time, I had nothing to fear (I didn't think) heartwise. I figured this was either a bad indigestion, or more likely, when I lifted weights, I may have pulled a muscle or perhaps held my breath as I lifted a heavy set of weights. At least, to me, this seemed like a more likely scenario than a heart problem. I don't think that I had this pain for at least a couple of weeks after this event. So I forgot about it.

By the second week of October, the same thing happened. I had that exact same pain again. I recall even mentioning it to a couple of people at work, but again in a couple of hours, it went away. Up until now, I had been working out on a regular basis running every third day, lifting every third day, and doing thirty to forty-five minutes on a stair stepper every third day, and was averaging six days a week working out. I was also noticing that the pain only occurred after I lifted weights.

In the last week of October, I took my family on a weeklong vacation to Florida, at Disney World. I don't travel well, and I don't particularly like vacations. They are stressful to me. But we stayed there for a week, took a plane both ways. And because my darling brother Jason was down there for a couple of days with me, I was "forced" to go on some of the scariest rides they have, including the Tower of Terror. This is like an elevator fall from fifteen or twenty stories. I went on roller coasters and really didn't avoid any rides. I had no pain at all in my chest, although my stomach was in knots due to the anxiety and stress from the trip itself.

After I got back from vacation, it was time for casino night. This was a church project for which I was the chairman of the board. It was a fund-raiser for the Catholic school that our children attended. It took a lot of work and coordination, and there was stress that accompanied this glorious job, but I still never had any pains or heart problems from this. The event occurred on November 6, 1999. We didn't make any money on the project, but everyone that attended had fun.

As I went through November and December, I had a couple of bouts with this burning chest pain. I still didn't worry about it because I knew that I could run four miles, do a stair stepper for forty-five minutes, and feel no pain. When I lifted weights, the pain would sometimes occur. Still I didn't like doctors, and I still didn't have a primary physician, and I knew that even if I was feeling good, a doctor would probably find something wrong with me anyway. I survived Thanksgiving and Christmas with no chest pains from stress and anxiety at all, just from the lifting of weights.

We have a family reunion at Saratoga Springs, New York, every other year. Up there, we drink a lot and eat a lot of food that can be bad for you. We did a little bowling and touch football. With all the stress a family reunion can bring, as well as the light athletics, I was fine. I should also mention that my lovely wife Sue had suffered from pneumonia from December 20 through January 10 or so. So I was in full charge of the children and taking care of her for the ending of 1999 and the beginning of 2000. We didn't have a lot of snow during the winter, perhaps a couple of three to four inch snows, but I shoveled them with ease. Let's get to the events of January 25 and 26. And again up until now, I had no clue what this pain was, just that it occurred only sometimes after I lifted weights.

I recall we had some snow on January 25 as well as some freezing rain that changed to plain rain. I went to work as usual, and there might have been two inches of slushy snow before it was all over. I asked my son, Chris, to shovel the driveway if he wanted to, and to my surprise he did it—not to my specs, but not too bad. When I got home at 7:30 or 8:00 p.m., I cleaned up the driveway a little bit and noticed that Chris did not shovel the front walkways at all. I wasn't upset, because I was dealing with an eleven-year-old child, an intelligent one, but I did say driveway. So I shoveled the front walks. I was finished within a half hour, and it was not physically demanding at all.

CHAPTER 10

The Actual Heart Attack and Hospital Stay

That night, I went to bed as usual. I usually get up two or three o'clock to use the bathroom. This night was no different. I woke up but noticed that I had a hint of that burning chest pain, but by the time I got back to bed, it had subsided and I went to sleep as usual. When I woke up at approximately 6:30 a.m., I had the chest pain again, and this time it was worse. There was no throbbing or pressure, no jolts of pain going down my left arm or anything. But it did hurt, and it was very uncomfortable. I sat in bed a couple of minutes, thought about doing a stair stepper workout for about five seconds, perhaps working my way through it, then I thought this was a crazy idea. I was having chest pains. I tried to breathe deeply because I thought it would alleviate the pain, but it didn't. I washed up quickly, brushed my teeth, and thought for a minute. This pain had been a thorn in my side (chest) for months. The pain was now more intense than it had ever been before; more important to me was the fact that the pain was there and I had really done nothing to cause it. I just woke up! This was very troubling to me.

It was now about 7:00 a.m., so I decided that I had better make a trip to the emergency room at our local hospital. The first thing I did was to go out to the driveway and start my car. I noticed a bottle of aspirin in a seat compartment and took two of them, knowing if this was a heart problem, aspirin is highly recommended. I went back in the house, waving to a couple of neighbors along the way, as the car warmed up. It was probably only twenty or twenty-five degrees outside at this time, but I didn't feel like checking the thermometer. I told my wife that I was going to go to the emergency room, which was about a six- or seven- minute drive away. She said she would call 911. I said (note that I am a type a+++ personality) that I did not feel like sitting around the house for ten or twenty minutes when I know I can be there in six or seven minutes. I remember knowing that in a heart attack situation, seconds are critical. Then my wife said, "I will drive you," again I said no. By the time she got herself and the kids ready, I knew that it would be ten or fifteen minutes to wait anyway. I also felt but didn't say that I didn't feel like discussing this for ten or fifteen minutes either. So I left the house, got into my car, which was warmed up enough so I could scrape a peek hole in the ice on the front window about four inches wide and four inches long that would allow me to see at least a little bit as I drove to the hospital. The chest pain was holding its own at this time, not getting any better or worse. I tried to go through the path of least resistance and passed a yellow or red light at one point, but I would have challenged anyone to stop me the way I felt. When I got to the hospital, I saw three ambulances blocking the entrance to the emergency room parking lot. So I simply took a quick turn and drove in the exit to the parking lot; there was no stopping me now.

Having arrived at the emergency entrance, I had to find a nurse or doctor, so I walked around a couple of corners and found a desk with a couple of nurses standing around. I said that I am having chest pains. One of the nurses said, "That's not good," and immediately led me to a room about fifteen feet away from where we were standing.

She said, "Take off all your clothes."

I did promptly, and then I said, "Here is my insurance card."

Her immediate reply was, "Don't even think about that, lie or sit down on this bed."

By now four or five other people had arrived. They were plugging holes in me like there was no tomorrow.

They were sticking electrodes on me. And within five minutes, one guy who was looking at a heart monitor said, "You are having a heart attack."

Most people would have been frightened at hearing this, but for me, the whole experience seemed too surreal to be scary. It was almost like watching this unfold in the third person, like a book I remember reading. I was just concerned about when the pain would stop. It was such a terrible pain at this point. I wanted it fixed. One of the first questions they asked me was if I had aspirin.

I said, "Yes, I took two before I came in."

They said that was the smartest thing I could have done. As an aside, a lot of people asked me about the aspirin, and it is the general consensus among the medical community that taking aspirin is the smartest thing one can do under these circumstances. Chewing would have been better (I just swallowed). The dumbest thing I did was to drive myself to the hospital. However, I explained my reasoning to you before.

For the next several minutes, nurses were giving me nitroglycerin pills and morphine. They stuck this nitroglycerin pill under my tongue, and I recall how thirsty I was; it just stayed there. It was supposed to be absorbed quickly, but I think my mouth was too dry. I asked for water, but they said no because they didn't know what other treatments I would need. Then they asked me how bad the pain was, on a scale of 1 to 10. That is an interesting question. I can't really say what the pain was. It depends on what a 10 is, and I didn't know, so I said the pain was a 7 or 8 on a scale of 1 to 10.

I want to add just a word here about morphine. This is a great medication. I was nervous and, as a result, felt cold. I also felt very tense with all the things going on around me. When they put a shot of morphine into one of those plastic tubes that was connected to my arm, I felt great. It only took the better part of five to ten seconds to work. I felt better. I felt warm, calm and relaxed. The pain was still there to some extent, but I didn't mind, thanks to this great drug. It felt so good that I discovered why it is so hot on the black market.

It was about this time that Nurse Ratched came in. She came in with about ten sheets of paper in her hands and said, "We are conducting a study with this new clot-busting medicine."

I would receive all the medicine I would normally get, but this new medicine, or a placebo, would be given in addition. No one would know if it was a placebo. At this point, I had been in there perhaps twenty minutes, and I don't know if it was the morphine wearing off, but the pain persisted, and Nurse Ratched read on.

I finally stopped her and said, "When someone is having a heart attack, aren't seconds critical?" She said yes, so I said, "I don't care what it is, just let me sign the damn thing, but get going and do what you have to do." Then she left to do her thing.

Now the pain, probably due mostly to the morphine (because then I still had the nitro pill under my tongue), subsided to a 5 on a scale of 1 to 10. People are still running around like crazy. One guy came in and put a rubber glove on.

I asked politely, "What the hell are you doing?"

He said politely, "I am going to stick my hand up your ass, bend over and say, 'Ahhh.'"

I asked, "Why?"

He said because when they give me this concoction of clot-busting drugs, if there is any hint of blood in my rectum, I could bleed to death in minutes.

I said, "I'm sorry I asked."

I hate when doctors stick their hand up your butt and say "excuse me" twenty times. I just tell them do it and get it done and forget about it. If we had been in West Virginia, I think we would be legally married now.

I must have been in the hospital forty or forty-five minutes (I'm not sure because everything was moving very fast and I now had a lot of drugs in me). I remember asking where the clot-busting stuff was. A nurse said they are mixing it up in the other room. Finally, they arrived and gave me the medication. In the meantime, many nurses and doctors, but not the head doctor (he had some car problems), were passing through. But they were not looking at me; they were looking over my head. This was a little disturbing. They were talking to me but looking at what I thought was the ceiling. After a while, I caught on. All the monitors were over my head where all the doctors and nurses were looking.

About five minutes after the heavy-duty clot busters were in me, everyone except for one nurse had left. Did they give up hope? I asked a few times how I was doing, but no one gave a hint of how sick I really was. Did they not know, or were they afraid of lawsuits if they said the wrong thing?

This one nurse talked to me and said, "I guess I should tell you this [I thought, *Uh-oh*], there is a thing called a breakthrough that a lot of people experience after taking these clot busters."

She said that if this occurs, it is a good thing. She said that sometimes when the clot breaks up and clears through your arteries, the pain can actually get a lot worse before it gets better. She went on to say the worse this pain is, the better your outcome will likely be.

She told me this in passing, like it was an afterthought. At any rate, the pain was now a 4, and my wife and kids finally made it to my room. I think it was important for the kids to see me so they could see everything was okay and not just fear the words heart attack. We chatted for five minutes or so when all of a sudden, I was getting a different kind of pain. Now, it was a more throbbing, pressure-filled pain. I told the nurse that I was getting this pain, and she quickly got the wife and kids out of the room. I reminded my wife to call work and tell them I wouldn't be in today. Now it was my chance to find out what a 10 on a 1–10 scale meant (or at least a 9.5). The throbbing got worse and worse. I am thinking how glad I was that the nurse remembered to tell me about this breakthrough. If she didn't, I swear that I would have thought it was all over. At this point, she was treating me like I was a delivering mother. She kept saying, "Breathe, breathe, breathe."

The pain did get to a 9.5 or a 10, and it lasted for what felt like an hour (in actuality, it was maybe a couple of minutes). When it got better, the pain felt like a 2 or 3 on a scale of 1 to 10. Was it a 2 or 3, or was the other pain so severe that the scale changed, that I don't know, but I did feel much better.

By now the folks at the hospital felt as though they did all they could for me. And all in all, I feel they did a very good job; they saved my life. My wife, kids, and now my father were in my room—just in time to hear that they were going to send me to another hospital, in New Haven, about fifteen to twenty minutes away. They packed me up in one of those ambulance stretchers and sent me off to the other hospital with a sheet (not over my head), in an ambulance with the lights and sirens on.

After having a brief conversation about golf with my ambulance nurse, I finally arrived in my new digs. They wheeled me directly into the cardiac care section, stuck me on an operating table (or should I say, slithered me from the ambulance stretcher to the operating table). There I lay, while looking at two TV sets with my name on them. These guys were waiting for me. They explained that they were going to do a cardiac cauterization—no balloon, just to see what was going on. So I signed forms that said basically it's okay if I died. Then they shaved my groin area, carefully, but a good part of my well-earned pubic hair was gone. Then they gave me a local anesthetic (like novocaine) and waited a minute. They cut a small hole into the femoral artery—not in my leg, but in my lower abdomen about as close to the leg as you can get, an inch or so above the leg. Once you feel the novocaine needle, you feel no other pain. Next thing you know, with the aid of some high-tech camera or ultrasound perched right over your chest, you are seeing your heart on TV. Really cool, although I wished I could watch someone else's heart on TV for obvious reasons.

I could hear the doctors talking to each other. It couldn't have been in English. It was some form of pig Latin that doctors invented just so they know that the patient does not understand what the hell they are talking about. My main doctor and some Indian doctor (from India, not America) kept shooting this dye into my heart and looking at the blood flow, doctors talk just like they write. When they finished the procedure, the nearest I could figure was that the artery was 40 percent clogged and they were planning to wait forty-eight hours and allow the clot to break up a little more; then they would do a balloon angioplasty to fully clear the artery and put in a stent. A stent is a wire-meshed tube that is designed to keep an artery open once it is cleared. I never heard how blocked the artery was during the actual attack. I also never found out what separates the other pains I had been having for months from the heart attack. Were these other pains small heart attacks or just warnings? I also never found out why the chest pains occurred only when lifting weights, not when running or stair-stepping. But let's move on.

After this first operation, they decided not to stitch me up. They placed a bandage over the opening and told me to do two things. Lie flat; don't even lift your head. And hold this bandage on the opening as hard as you can. I thought this was quite a responsibility. I just had a heart attack. I was full of blood thinners. My femoral artery was just opened, and I had to hold a bandage over the opening so

I wouldn't bleed to death. Just what was I paying for, anyway? I do think they were concerned about blood loss, but there should be a better technique than just having the patient apply direct pressure.

What seemed to be five hours was more likely forty-five minutes. Someone in the recovery room looked at my wound and said that I had a rather large hematoma. I never saw it. I never even looked or wanted to see it. But finally a doctor put on a device, I don't know what it is called, that basically just squeezes the wound and puts enough pressure on the area (it was on for hours) to stop the bleeding. Eventually, it worked. The next problem was their inability to find a room right away, so I was stuck in this recovery room for about three hours on my back, not lifting my head. Try this sometime. My chest hurt just from that, with still some minor pain lingering from the heart attack. It got down right uncomfortable. After three hours, I received a change of scenery. I was moved to a private room in the ICU, the intensive cardiac care unit. This was class. There was even a TV in there. But for the first three hours, the nurses were very insistent that I would not move and still had to keep flat in bed. This was to assure that I would not bleed again. I admit I cheated quite a bit as time went on. Really, at this point, bleeding to death didn't seem like such a bad alternative.

While I was in the intensive care unit, my mother (God bless her) began to bug me. Apparently, she talked to one of the doctors, and one of them must have told her about my one bad habit. She asked me why I chewed tobacco. She started screaming, ranting, and raving. I, in the meantime, had some problems of my own with which I was trying to deal. I had chest pains. I had a heart attack. I had all kinds of drugs. I also had a small thing, like a major heart operation. Oh, yeah, I also had to lie on my back and hold a hole in my femoral artery so I wouldn't bleed to death. All in all, I was pretty much defenseless. Now I had to keep my anxiety down and blood pressure low. Try not to get stressed while this maniac of a woman screamed her head off at me. I love my mother; of course, she had her reasons and was extremely worried. Ninety percent of the time, she is a very nice person. I just happened to catch her when she exploded from her deep concern. The good news is that my sister Jill had pointed all this out to her, and then she agreed perhaps she was being too overwhelming at this point, thought the better of it, and apologized and didn't scream at me for at least week.

That evening, the device finally came off. The nurses must have had strict orders to check out the groin area for swelling or hematoma (either that or they just wanted to check out my black-and-blue penis) because they must have checked out the site every half hour or so.

Let me explain for a brief moment about my genitalia being black and blue. At some time during this ordeal—I really can't remember when, everything was moving so fast at this point—one of the doctors, or nurses, thought it would be great fun to stick this device on my penile area. I guess, in the long term, it would save many trips to the bathroom. All in all, it is preferable to a catheter. This thing is a plastic attachment that holds a rubber tube that goes into a bag so you can pee without going to the bathroom. It fits on the end of a penis like a tight balloon. The only problem with this device is that I believe it was held on by superglue. There is no way in this world it is coming off. After several days in the hospital, before I was about to leave, I took it off—suffice it to say it wasn't easy. This would be funny if it didn't happen to me. After all was said and done, my penis was black and blue. This would have been great if I was black, but one could easily tell it wasn't big enough. I will allude to this later, but for now, I just want you to know how it became it black and blue.

I still had some chest pain at that time, but I didn't know if this pain was the result of lying flat on my back for six hours (that would always cause non–heart-related chest discomfort for me) or residual heart attack pain. As the evening wore on, the nurse kept asking how the pain felt, and I was saying it was a 2 or 3 on a scale of 1 to 10. It wasn't bad, but it was there, and it was annoying. By about midnight, the nurse said that the doctors decided to do the angioplasty twenty-four hours early. They would perform this operation on Thursday instead of Friday. After that, I rested comfortably all night, one of the best nights of sleep I have had in a long time. *Yeah*! If you believe that I have some beach front land in Arizona I would like to sell you. For the money these hospitals charge, you would think they would make it easier to sleep, especially when you have just had a heart attack. One would think sleep would be the best thing for you. I had three IVs in my arms, about twenty to twenty-five sticky pads on me so they could hook up their EKG machines. They had a blood pressure cuff on my arm that was automatic. A person was not needed to pump it up; since it was timed. It would pump up my arm at the exact time I would just start to doze off. With all the wires attached to these sticky pads and the IVs and the pressure cuff, you could not move in bed; you were stuck on your back. The only real adjusting you could do was with the elevation of the bed. The sun came up, and an Oriental nurse came in the room. I thought she was going to start prepping me for the operation, but no, she had a better assignment. She had to look at the veins in my neck and measure how long they were. Don't ask me why she never told me, and I was afraid to ask.

About 7:30 a.m., they took me down to the cardiac operating room, the same one I had been in the morning before. The first thing I had to do was to sign another form that said that if I had a stroke or blood clot or if I died for any reason, it would be my fault. They had the same two TVs hooked up with my name showing. There the same two doctors (my doctor and the same Indian doctor) prepping to do the surgery. They gave a drug to relax me but again kept me awake during the operation. They decided to operate on the other side of my lower stomach (femoral artery area), which made me very happy because the other side hurt like hell from the day before. One nurse warned me that when they inflate the balloon, it may feel like I was having a heart attack again for a brief time. This got me a little nervous, but it never did feel like the heart attack pain during the surgery. One of the doctors shot novocaine in the area, and once again, before I knew it, the probe was in my heart.

This operation, in my mind, should have taken about half an hour. It actually took two and a half hours because of all the talking and bickering everyone was doing in the operating room. For instance, they kept telling me how big my arteries were. They said I have huge arteries. I still didn't know if this is a good thing to have. I was hoping and assuming they were big from all the exercise I had always done, but on the other hand, it must have been a large blood clot if it closed up a huge artery. At any rate, they went up the artery and inserted the balloon device into the proper spot. They inflated it a few times, but I felt nothing. I would like to know what happens to pieces of clot that are broken off and shot through your arteries. Can it cause another heart attack or stroke? I was afraid to ask, so I never found out. The funniest, and scariest, part of this operation came when they were putting the stent in. Studies have shown that vessels opened by the balloon tend to close up again in laboratory mice. I guess, for now, I am a laboratory mouse.

Next, I heard my doctor ask for a number 6 stent. Then I heard a nurse say, "We don't have any number 6s. The biggest we have is a 5."

Then I realized it was probably a disadvantage to have huge arteries.

But the doctor had a solution. He said, "We will use a chubby 5," whatever that is.

I think they overexpand a 5 and call it a chubby 5. It seemed to sound good to the crew, even though it scared the hell out of me. So after what seemed to be forever, they got their chubby 5 stent, and I guess it was the Indian doctor who was guiding the stent into place and my doctor was telling him where to put it.

He was saying things, like, "A little further," "No, take it back," "A little more," "A little more," "Okay perfect."

Then I heard these infamous words I will never forget, and I quote, "Okay, let's not burst anything."

I almost asked him to repeat this, but it might have made him burst something. After they changed my underwear and calmed me down, they assured me that they didn't burst anything. At this point, the operation was almost over. One of the nurses said that there was one test they wanted to do and warned me that I would feel a warm rush throughout my body when they put in this dye as it flushed through. It was weird but not overall a bad thing. I guess they were using ultrasound equipment because just before they were finished, one nurse asked me if I had to pee. I said, "Like a racehorse."

She said, "Your bladder is twice the size it should be, why don't you pee now?"

I said, "I'm gun-shy. I was planning to do it as soon as I got out of here," remembering I still had that tube on, but I at least wanted a little privacy. It was finally time to finish the operation.

I don't know if the original novocaine wore off, but I remember the doctors had a short discussion and decided to stitch up the wound this time. Remember that they did not stitch up the one from the previous day, and there was some sort of a hematoma. So they injected me with novocaine again, and it hurt again. The doctors waited an appropriate time, about ten seconds, and started stitching. Believe me, I felt everything; this was the worst part of the operation. I was squirming around, telling the doctor that I had a great idea: "Let's wait a few minutes and let the novocaine take effect."

The only comment I heard from the Indian doctor was, "Sorry, sorry, sorry," but he just kept on going.

He must have had a date. He didn't slow down a bit. Eventually, the ordeal was over. I wasn't paying attention, but by this point, all the chest pain had finally subsided, probably because the lower abdominal pain was worse. As soon as I hit the recovery room, I waited for a private moment and pissed for what seemed like ten minutes.

This time I was in the recovery room for only a half an hour or so, and they took me up to my room once again. They said that after lying on my back (but not as flat as the first day), I would be getting out of bed later that afternoon or in the evening. As we went to my room, I was accompanied by the Indian doctor. I asked him after doing all the tests and operations what kind of damage was done by this heart attack. He said, in as vague terms as possible, that my heart was 30 to 35 percent less efficient now than it was before the heart attack. I thought he must be kidding me because I didn't feel that bad. He said it was very hard to say exactly what the real damage was because much of the damage could be caused by the shock of the attack. Some heart function would return back, but there was no way of saying how much would come back. To skip ahead for a minute, when my doctor talked to me the next morning, he said that the Indian doctor might have been too optimistic in assessing the damage. He said it was more, like, 45 to 50 percent damaged. But again, some function would come back, but no one knew just how much. I still didn't believe this figure.

It was Thursday afternoon. Lots of people visited me: Mom, Dad, in-laws, and outlaws. I was feeling a little tired but all in all pretty good, considering what I had been through. My two brothers and sister were with me in the room. The nurse came in (Mike was his name), and he inserted something into one of my IV tubes. I asked what this was for.

He said, "To clean you out from all the dye they put into you during the operation."

I said, "I'll be pooping all afternoon?"

He said, "No, more like peeing."

Since I am camera shy, or gun-shy, or whatever, I had to kick my brothers and sister out of the room four or five times during the next hour so I could pee. I must have urinated a gallon in that hour, all through that tube. Sometimes peeing is better than sex. This was one of those times, but you would barely finish peeing and the family would come back, and in five minutes, that urge was back; it was very embarrassing.

After this was done, Mike allowed me to take my peeing tube off. I think he was trying to be nice. I guess he knew it would hurt a little. And he told me that he didn't like doing it himself; it was less painful if I did it myself. I think letting me do it made both of us feel a little more comfortable. It didn't hurt a lot, but when I looked at "King Kong," that is what my wife calls it (some girls call it, the penis, longata), it was black. I assumed that it must have been some glue residue. After I got home, even after several very intense washings, it was still black. It was black for a good two weeks after that. I still don't know exactly why. Was it from the massive black-and-blues I had from the two operations in the groin area, or did the tube create its own black-and-blue? I guess I will never know.

Late that afternoon, my male nurse Mike came in and set up a chair for me to sit in. He didn't let me walk yet; he was afraid that I would fall. When I got out of bed for the first time, I realized how much pain (not heart pain, groin pain) there was. The only thing that I recall even coming close to this pain was when I had my hernia operation back in 1972 (when I had to fake pissing to be released). It really felt like they sewed my leg to my stomach. But this time, they did it on both sides of my body. Needless to say, I was moving very, very slowly. It was about 7:00 p.m. when the nurse finally let me walk around the floor. Boy, was this painful, but I just trudged along. It was at this time that I realized that there were some sick people in here. I mean, people lying in bed with the TV off (that alone means they are really sick to me). They had oxygen masks on, tubes all over their bodies, with that all-too-familiar hospital gray color. Some hardly moving, some struggling to breathe—it was a nasty wake-up call to reality. I, all of a sudden, realized that with all the pain I was in, I still was easily the luckiest (healthiest) one on the floor. Here I was, taking a nice romantic walk with the nurse, and one of the nurses on the floor said to me, "Boy, we don't get too many walkie-talkies on this floor."

Later, on that same walk, another nurse near my room, caught me walking with the nurse, and said, "What are you doing?"

It may have been the drugs, but I replied, "I'm a 'walking cutie,'" which made everyone laugh.

That night I slept better than the previous night. I do recall at one point pulling all the wires off my chest because I couldn't turn over in bed. I thought these wires had been used for an EKG or other tests they did several hours earlier and they forgot to disconnect them. But about two minutes after I did this, the nurse came in and said, "Are you okay?"

I said, "Sure, I'm a walking cutie."

She told me my monitor on the front desk indicated I was dead. I said, "Oops," and explained what I did, so she had to hook me up again.

Other than that, it was a fairly eventless night. The next day, Friday, I was about to move. Everyone said I was going to go home on Saturday, and I would have preferred to stay put for one more day, but they needed the bed, I guess. So I went to a less intense area of the hospital—or at least, that is what they told me—and by midaft- ernoon Friday, I was in my new digs.

Just a quick note on the "faking a piss" comment in the previous paragraph. I should explain that back in 1972, I developed a hernia. After the operation to repair the hernia, I was all set to go home. The hospital said that I couldn't be released until I urinated. I didn't have the urge to urinate, but I did have the urge to go home. I went into the bathroom, and there was a small water pitcher there. I filled it up and slowly poured it into the toilet bowl and moaned like some people do when they pee. It worked, so I went home. Circa 1980, something, somehow my operation was being discussed, and I told my mother about this. She got really mad at me for doing this. I was probably thirty at the time; what was she mad at? I told her that I have peed since, so everything worked out fine, even though I faked it.

I was no longer in a private room, and as nice and comfortable as my old room was, this one was equally uncomfortable. There was a seventy-year-old guy next to me who did nothing but cough and talk to himself. He would cough and yell at the nurses to get him a cough drop. They never did, and he would keep whining, "Oh, I'm so tired, I wish I could sleep," "I can't stop coughing," "I am so tired, oh my god."

Wow, I can understand some complaining, but when all is said and done, I was too sick too to listen to his problems. I needed rest, and this room was probably cost $2,000-$3,000 a day at this price I shouldn't have to put up with this nonsense. I didn't need this stuff. It was a constant thing; he would not shut up. After I was in this room for about an hour or two, I took a walk. As I returned to my highly priced room, a nurse greeted me at the door and said that they were having a problem with my roommate and asked if I could stay out of the room for a while. At this point, I was just hoping he was not contagious. I had all my visitors that evening in the lounge near my room. I couldn't even lie down unless it was on a couch. I had to eat there, and I was getting very agitated because they sent me to this visiting area instead of my room. After all my guests left around 9:00 p.m. or so, I still couldn't go back to my room.

I finally returned at about 9:30 p.m. I was greeted at the door by this box containing 5-liter jars of this yellowish fluid (the way the food tasted in this place, I am sure they probably used it and called it chicken soup Saturday evening). A nurse said they had taken this fluid out of my roommate's chest. I heard someone later describe how much fluid was in him by saying that you could hear his clavicle creaking when he moved. Why didn't anyone pick up on this earlier (I smell lawsuit)? As I tried to go to sleep around 10:30 or 11:00 p.m., I noticed that the guy was still talking to himself. I realized he felt better because he was now griping about how thirsty he was. Every time a shadow would pass the door, he would beg for ice cubes. Every time no one was around, he moaned, "I'm tired, I'm thirsty, I have to pee, etc." I could not catch a break from this guy.

Finally, he began to shut up around 1:00 a.m. I was just dozing off when I heard a nurse (a male nurse with a *loud* Southern voice) wake up this guy (and I) to tell him his blood pressure was too low. I was thinking, *Let him die already, at least he will be quiet.* (Just kidding.) I know it sounds very mean, but I tried to get him some help. I tried to find my nurse to ask for a couple of sleeping pills, which finally arrived an hour later. I probably got a total of an hour of sleep that night. No one told me that a heart attack could be so much fun.

Finally, daybreak—the sun was rising, birds were chirping, the guy next to me was dead, this is great (only kidding about the guy next to me). And the nurse informed me that I would be able to leave at about 10:00 a.m. I couldn't wait.

My wife was late picking me up, but I didn't even scream at her. I saw a young kid wheeling a wheelchair down the hall, and it became apparent that he was my ticket out of the hospital. He was a small kid, weighing no more than 70 lbs. soaking wet, about thirteen or fourteen years old. But in the four or five minutes I was with him, he impressed me. He was very talkative and bright.

At the start, I said, "Are you going to make it?" Because I was three times his size.

Of course, he said yes. My wife was impressed because he got her parking ticket stamped, so she parked free when she picked me up. She used to like these simple pleasures, not anymore.

CHAPTER 11

My Return Home

After an uneventful trip, I finally arrived home. We pulled in to my driveway, which was covered with two inches of solid ice, and there was nothing I could do about it. Sure, someone could have shoveled it when it was soft, but I don't think napalm would help now. I did the penguin walk to the house; it would have been hard to walk under normal conditions on this ice, but when they sew both of your legs to your stomach, it makes it that much more challenging.

After my walk across the ice, I put on some freshly laundered underpants. The first thing I wanted to do was take a shower. It was Saturday now, and the last time I took one was on Tuesday morning. I am sure I smelled like last week's garbage. Remember, doctors told me that I had 30 to 50 percent damage to the heart. To be honest, I didn't believe them. I have been exercising all my life, and I know that I could have run five miles on Tuesday, and I knew that even with four days off, I could still run five miles. You simply don't get out of shape so quickly. In the hospital I was untested. The most activity I could do was walk down a hall. I must admit that reality hit when I walked up my first flight of stairs. I was actually winded (not huffing and puffing like there was no tomorrow), but it was definitely much harder to walk up one flight of stairs then I could ever remember it being. At that point, I really knew something was wrong. That was shock number 1.

Next, I very slowly and gingerly took off my clothes to take a shower. I then looked in the mirror to see the scope of the black-and-blue areas on me. From my belly button to the bottom of my groin, I was black and blue. It was weird, but judging from the pain I experienced, the black-and-blues were proportional. I also found several more sticky pads that the nurses somehow forgot to take off in the hospital. I believe that even a week later, I found one near the rib cage on the side. I'm glad I didn't go to the beach; it would have looked really stupid. I slowly took my shower; it felt good to finally be semiclean. I remember washing and scrubbing my penis to see if it was glue or black and blue. It was black and blue (I still occasionally scrub it but for different reasons). I stopped scrubbing after a certain point because with all the blood thinners, I figured it would only get worse.

It was time to start my new life—no more tobacco. If I ever become terminally ill, that is the first habit I will start again, however. By the way, have you ever noticed that there are no good habits that are fun and enjoyable? For instance, people smoke or chew tobacco. It feels good, and we like it, but it is not good for you. People drink, but it is not good for you. The only exception to this rule is we can drink wine, but only in small amounts. Think about it, and try to find one good habit that feels good and is fun and is good for you. There is not one I can think of. People do drugs; it feels good, but it is not good for you. People work out (this is a good habit) but it sucks to exercise. This is how life goes. Were you to survive a would-be nuclear holocaust and all books and doctors are vaporized, if you want to live a long and healthy life but you don't know how, use the Joe test. If it feels good, don't do it; if it feels or tastes like crap, do it and you will live forever.

It's on to my new life. I remember talking with the nutritionist at the hospital. I couldn't chew tobacco, take more than one caffeine beverage per day (and I do love Coke!), eat very little fat, and the least amount of salt possible. Oh, and have fun doing it, and don't worry too much. I quickly learned, by reading labels, how to do this. There was not too much fat and salt in things like pasta and bread products. Great, so until my first doctor's appointment, this is what I ate, along with numerous salads. This worked out okay until the doctor ordered a blood test and found my triglycerides were going through the roof. No one told me this would happen. So he gave me a new prescription, Tricor, which would lower these nasty things. Triglycerides are fatty deposits that are in your blood, but somehow different from cholesterol, which was okay on this blood test.

I said, "If these drugs do exist, can I please have enough of them so I can have a Sausage McMuffin a couple of times a week?"

Now I have new rules: no tobacco, no caffeine, no fat, no salt, no carbs, no anything. I am going to turn into a rabbit. I am sure that in a couple of weeks, doctors will declare salads no good. I am thinking, *Why did I have to survive this thing?* Eating after a heart attack is a fate worse than death. Oh, I forgot, sugar is a carb, so no sugar or honey either.

During the first week at home, my mother and sister and the entire family were very nice to me as well as always accessible. One of them would come every day just to chat and, most of all, cook. They would buy the food they cooked, and they would cook tasty healthy meals that they practically invented using their sugar busters cook-book, which is another in a long line of controversial books about which some say are good then change their minds again.

My mom, bless her heart, at seventy years old, was the one who finally cleared the ice from my driveway. She was too weak to shovel and chop it, so every day she would throw a healthy amount of sand and rock salt on the driveway, and after one week, it was clear. That lowered my blood pressure by about forty points. Within a week, my mother and I and my niece Ella went to the Price Club to buy a snowblower. I love to shovel, but if I can't, and if I do have to buy a snowblower, I am going to get a good one, the Binford 6100. When in doubt, overkill was my motto. I ended up buying a huge 10-horse-power blower. I have seen too many people suffer with snow brooms and blowers that can handle only one type of fluffy snow. If the snow wasn't right, the snowblowers actually made it harder to remove than shoveling would have. This caused two problems. First of all, it was so big that to fit it in my mother's Land Rover, we had to flatten all the seats except for the front two. Did I mention my niece came with us? My mother, who can be very persistent like the immovable force, refused to drive anywhere because Ella would have to sit on my lap—that is, no seatbelt. I said, "Just go to my house" (it was about fifteen miles away), and I assured her nothing would happen. She wouldn't. She called Ella's mother, my sister, and told her to come and pick up Ella so she could take the snowblower to my house. After an hour's wait, we drove to my house where problem number 2 was waiting. There was no one to help take the snowblower out of the Land Rover. I could have, but my mom and wife said no way. It was time to get some favors from the past returned. You will see in the next paragraph why, but I had a friend named Tom, who answered the call. I helped him out a couple of years earlier. He single-hand-edly got the snowblower out of the Land Rover.

There was one year, three to four years before the heart attack, where I would shovel many driveways. That year was bad; we had about 100 to 120 inches of snow. I remember that I always had to shovel my driveway, then my neighbor's driveway, because they were old enough to fart dust. Then the lady across the street needed a path from her garage to her mailbox; she was old and widowed. For years, this was my normal snowstorm routine, but Tom had taken this year (the worst snow year in fifty years) to have a hernia, so I walked a block away and shoveled his very steep hilly driveway whenever it snowed. I was usually dead tired when it snowed because of all this shoveling. It was payback time, and we finally had a snowstorm. I think it was my third week home. I had my snowblower now, so I was not too worried when it snowed. I made a deal with the neighbor across the street, a mechanical-type guy. The deal was that was he could use the snowblower if he did my driveway.

One day we had about six to eight inches of snow, and being a weatherman, I knew it would change to sleet and freezing rain at night. I knew from previous experiences that I did not want to shovel this snow until the entire storm was over. It is much easier to remove snow with ice on top of it than it is to remove the snow and have an inch of freezing rain and sleet right on the pavement. This night my neighbor came over, and I suggested that he use the snowblower to do his front walk. I also said don't do my driveway. He didn't, so I dodged bullet number 1. I looked out the window at about 8:00 p.m. and caught my next-door neighbor starting to do my driveway (I guess everyone feels sorry for the heart attack guy). I begged him to stop, which he did. So I dodged bullet number 2. At about 9:00 p.m., my wife yelled for me (her voice could crack glass sometimes) and said that Tom is shoveling, but when I saw him, he was halfway finished, so I didn't bother to stop him. I didn't dodge bullet number 3 and, of course, paid the consequences the next day—not by cleaning the ice, because no one would let me, but by admiring the ice.

The rest of my recovery was going great for the first couple of weeks. I should say that I had a total of just over four weeks off from work due to the heart attack from Wednesday, January 26, 2000 (the date of the heart attack), until Friday February 25. I do think that I should have disconnected my phone line because the phones were ringing more at home than they were at work. I hate phones. You start feeling like Pavlov's dogs after a while. The bell rings; you have to do something. I do like caller ID, though, at least you don't have to talk to any annoying salesmen.

I didn't mention what happened to my brother Jason, the brother I didn't want around for my heart attack. It is not that I didn't want him around, but he lives in Florida and he had to fly to Connecticut for this—which means that when he has his heart attack, I have to go to Florida, and I don't travel well. On his flight back, he had to stop in Charlotte, North Carolina; and on his way there, lightning struck his plane. No real damage, but it was one loud bang accompanied simultaneously by a bright flash. I told him I caused it.

It was nice to be home. I wish I could qualify for my long-term disability and stay there, but finally, the time came to go to work. Before I explain how bad that was, let me tell you that even though I was home with a heart attack—to at least some degree caused by the clients I had to deal with—three clients had the nerve to call me at home during my first week or two there. I didn't want to talk to these people. These are the same people who contributed to my heart attack. Do you think I want to hear from them when I'm home? I didn't enjoy that part of my stay at home because I felt like I was at work. When I got back to work, I have to admit, the first few hours were not bad. But much as I explained the weather a couple hundred times a day, now I had to explain my heart attack. I dislike hypocrites. First they say, "Gee, how are you, what happened? Are you better, blah, blah, blah," then they start grilling you on, "Will it rain on my parade on Sunday?" I would like to make it a federal law that people at work can't tell anyone when someone else is sick. There is too much time wasted on your personal life. If the company says no personal calls, then you shouldn't mix pleasure (personal information) on business calls. I tell people that I don't socialize with clients because it would affect my decision-making, just like a brain surgeon. It sounds like a great excuse anyway.

At this point in my life, I am working and trying to eat right. I haven't started rehab yet, so my workouts are limited to walking very briskly up and down a hill, which is a one and a half mile course around my house. I had a couple of uneventful appointments with my cardiologist. I will likely have some good stories perhaps in another book. I have had one stress test so far. Here is a thing that bothered me about that. I went in to the hospital to take this test. Two nurses were operating this equipment for the stress echocardiogram. They take pictures of your heart with ultrasound, as they do with pregnant mothers. They take one set before you get stressed on a treadmill. The nurses did this. While we were waiting for the doctor to show up and actually test me, they had my heart movie (tape) going.

I asked, "How does it look?"

The nurse, the more experienced of the two, said, "I'm not the doctor."

I said, "I could see that, but I know you have seen a few thousand more of these things than I have."

She said, "I'm not the doctor."

I said, "So you know, but you are afraid to tell me." I said, "Look, I'm not going to sue you or hold anything against you, but instead of saying nothing in this fifteen minutes waiting for the doctor, we can talk."

This really loosened her up. She said that by looking at the tape, she could tell that I had had a heart attack. I knew we were finally getting somewhere.

So I asked, "How?"

She said, "I am not the doctor."

After going through this browbeating and trying to draw blood from a stone, I got her to point to a small section on the screen and say, "This part of the heart wall is not moving as much as that part."

It was at this point I figured I better shut up and consider myself lucky for the information I received already. This woman should have been handed our biggest national secrets and then tortured by the Vietnamese to see if she would crack; they would have shot her out of frustration. The doctor finally showed up, and we continued the test that would consist of nine minutes on the treadmill.

Three minutes easy, three minutes moderate, and three minutes hard. He asked after the three minutes easy, "Are you tired?"

I said no. He was insulting me. After five minutes, "No, but I am getting a little winded and huffing a little."

Tired is a terrible word to use. I could have gone on at this pace forever. The final three minutes were harder, but little challenge to get through. They took their movie under stress successfully. Then the doctor started talking all this doctor talk with this nurse. "Oh, this is bigger than before," he then said. "This is classic, star this frame."

After a few minutes, at least the doctor had the courtesy to say all the stuff we are talking about is good news. That is all I got out of him. I tried to get more out of him, so I asked some questions, and all he could say is that the test indicated that the heart disease that I had in that one bad artery didn't seem to be occurring in other arteries.

He said, "Try to start the rehab."

I said, "I did, but there is a waiting line." I said, "Could I run or lift or do anything in the meantime?"

He said, "No, try to do the rehab first."

I asked if and when could I have sex.

He said, "You could have it anytime you want, but only do it with your wife, I don't want you to get too excited."

So here I am right now. I'm just waiting for rehab. But no chest pain at the present.

CHAPTER 12

The Moral of the Story

Well, the way I see it, when you are born, your heart has a certain number of beats given to it. It varies from person to person. No one knows how many beats you have. No study can show this, and doctors won't admit this is the case either. Or else, they would be out of a job. But no matter what you do, even through exercise, you can't get more beats. As a matter of fact, I recommend not exercising because you will use up your limited number of beats faster than if you sat on the couch and ate potato chips. I often think back on all the times the boys wanted to go drinking or partying and I said, "No, I have to lift weights." Or that Florida vacation at spring break, waking up at 5:00 a.m. to run for two hours, how stupid. Not only did it take some fun away; it shortened my life. I say, be fat, eat what you want, drink all you want, take advantage of all those bad habits. I don't think it will make a difference. Let's suppose I am wrong. I challenge anyone to explain my heart attack at forty-three years of age. It's possible to walk out in the street and get hit by a bus tomorrow. Does it really make a difference? To take an extreme case, I can give you a 1000 percent guarantee that in seventy to eighty years, none of this will matter. In the end, I guess this whole mess is my wife's fault. She was with me every step of the way and I am convinced she is bad luck. Happy thoughts!

Other morals if you stretch your imagination are the following:

It's not how long you make it; it's how you make it long.

When you go to kiss your honey, and her nose is kinda runny, you might think it's funny, but it's not.

Never speak badly about someone unless you walk a mile in their shoes. This way, when you do say something, you are a mile away and you got their shoes.

OTHER BOOK TITLES

Sitting under the Bleachers, by Seymour Butts
The Hawaiian Sex Book, by Komoni Wantolayya
Fraternities, by Fi Masta Beta Kow
Sexually Transmitted Diseases, by Ivan Cockburn
100 Yards to the Outhouse, by Willie Maikit,
illustrated by Betty Won't
Chest Pain, by I. Coffalot
Small Treasures in the Toilet Bowl, by I. P. Nickels
The German Bank Robbery, by Hans Zupp
Baby's Revenge, by Nora Titoff
Infectious Diseases, by Willie Catchlt
The Moons of Saturn, by Rosie Cheeks
Tigers Revenge, by Claude Balls
Inside Neverland Ranch, by Holden and Sharon Dix
How to Meet a Woman, by Heywood Jablomey

About the Author

The author's name is Joe Mauro, and this is a story that is 100 percent true. The heart attack occurred in the year 2000, when he was forty-three years old. He is one of five children who were born in Staten Island, New York. As a family, they moved to Connecticut in 1968, where he lived through high school. He has two bachelor of science degrees: one from Southern Connecticut State College, in physical education. He graduated in 1979. The other was a degree at the University of Oklahoma that he received in 1984 in meteorology. Besides studying there, he chased tornadoes with Oklahoma University as well as with the National Severe Storms Laboratory in Norman, Oklahoma. He has seen a total of around forty tornados. He moved back to Connecticut in 1985. His main job from 1985 through 2000 was as a meteorologist for a major corporate and aviation meteorology company in White Plains, New York. It was a commute of about fifty miles each away from where he lived, through heavy traffic, which he was convinced was a contributing factor to the heart attack. You will find out about others as well as you read I Am Joe's Heart "Attack." If you have had half as much fun reading this book as he had presenting it, this means he had twice as much fun as you. Enjoy!

CPSIA information can be obtained
at www.ICGtesting.com
Printed in the USA
FFOW03n2354030217
31981FF

9 781684 099894